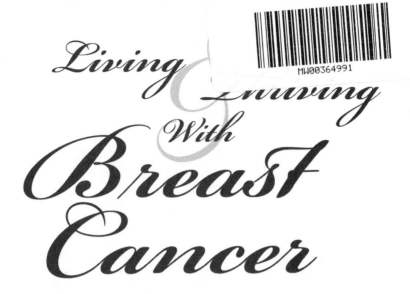

Living & Thriving With Breast Cancer

Stephanie Moline, MD
Joni Nichols, MD
Victor Gonzalez, MD
Saritha Thumma, MD
Robert K. Fairbanks, MD
Wayne T. Lamoreaux, MD
Jason A. Call, MD
Heather Gabbert, MS, RD, LD, CD
Tess Taft, MSW, LICSW
Kathy Beach, RN
Christopher M. Lee, MD

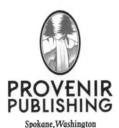

PROVENIR PUBLISHING

Spokane, Washington

The development of this patient handbook was sponsored by grants from:

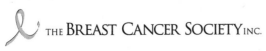

THE BREAST CANCER SOCIETY INC.

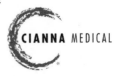

CIANNA MEDICAL

Living & Thriving With Breast Cancer

Published by Provenir Publishing, LLC, P. O. Box 211, Greenacres, WA 99016-0211

Production Credits

Lead Editor: Christopher Lee

Production Director: Micah Harman

Art Director and Illustration: Micah Harman

Cover Photo: Micah Harman

Printing History: June 2013, First Edition.

www.provenirpublishing.com

This book is dedicated to those breast cancer patients who inspire us every day as they climb the mountains they face.

Contents

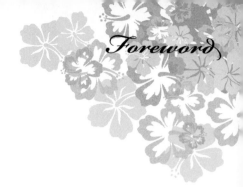

If you are reading this book, it is likely that you, a close family member, or close friend has been diagnosed with breast cancer. In most cases, this diagnosis was a shock. There are probably a 1000 questions floating around in your head; like how will this diagnosis be treated, how will you feel, how will this affect your family and your work, and what should you do next. Any cancer diagnosis has an impact on many aspects of life.

The goal of this book is to provide you with knowledge about your diagnosis and to assist in clarifying procedures, alleviate fears, and help you optimize your treatment. Our hope is that it also assists in alleviating anxiety as well as answering questions that commonly come up with a cancer diagnosis. In addition, we have included a section on practical nutritional techniques that can add to your ability to heal, improve your immune health, and optimize your energy and overall health.

Cancers of the breast affect patients in a wide variety of ways and, like other cancers, require a team of physicians and health care providers to assist in treatment.

This book is a compilation of experience and expertise that is easily interpreted. It is designed to provide rapid assistance in answering questions and guidance for you in your cancer journey.

Part One

What Is Breast Cancer?

Cancer cells originate from once normal cells within the body that have undergone genetic mutations leading to abnormal behavior. Breast cancer develops because of uncontrolled growth of abnormal cells within the breast. The growth and development of normal cells in our body are controlled and directed by genes primarily housed in the nucleus of the cell. Cancer develops when the normal genetic machinery directing the cells mutates, or changes, allowing uncontrolled growth. A breast cell with these mutations, grows and divides much more rapidly than the surrounding normal cells.

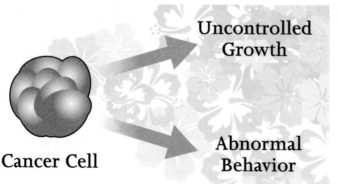

fig. 1.1

Cancer cells start with abnormal DNA.

It can take many years for some tumors (a collection of cancer cells) to be large enough to be detectable on an imaging study, such as a mammogram, or to be palpable. A 1 cm tumor (approximately ½ inch) can contain as many as one billion cancer cells.

Normal breast tissue is composed of lobules (where milk is produced), ducts (which carry the milk to the nipple complex), and fatty and connective tissue. Most often, breast cancer develops from the cells that line the duct (**ductal cancer**) or the lobule (**lobular cancer**). Rarely does cancer in the breast develop from the supportive structures.

fig. 1.2

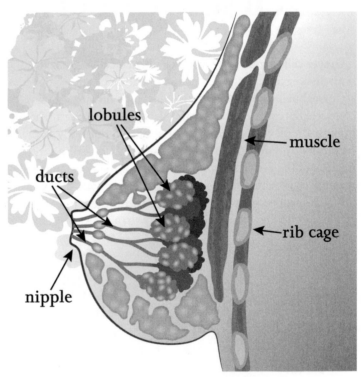

Anatomy of the breast.

Breast cancer can be divided into **2 general categories, non-invasive breast cancer** (or in situ cancer) and **invasive** (also known as infiltrating cancer). In situ cancer can develop in the lobule (LCIS or lobular carcinoma in situ) or the duct

(DCIS or ductal carcinoma in situ). Cancer cells grow and divide within these structures (lobules or ducts), but don't penetrate the wall of the structures and therefore do not gain access to other areas in the body. Invasive cancers, on the other hand, grow through the structure walls and/or into the surrounding tissues and through this have access to lymphatic channels and blood vessels which creates the potential to spread to other parts of the body. (see fig. 4.3, pg. 15)

Part Two

How Do I Know If I Have Breast Cancer? What Are The Common Causes?

Breast cancer is often found by a patient or caregiver identifying something that isn't "normal". This could be a distinct lump or a vague thickening, a change in skin color or texture, a change in nipple shape, or an abnormal nipple discharge. Breast cancer can also be discovered on a screening mammogram as a new asymmetrical solid density within the tissue, or as micro-calcifications (tiny calcium deposits).

What Are The Common Symptoms Of Breast Cancer?

It is important to understand that each person can have different symptoms leading to a diagnosis of breast cancer. In some women, breast cancer can be present without any symptoms. In women who undergo regular mammograms, breast cancers as small as a few millimeters can be found long before they would be felt by a woman or her physician. In these cases, the radiologist makes a recommendation for further imaging and then a biopsy if needed to clarify the situation.

fig. 2.1

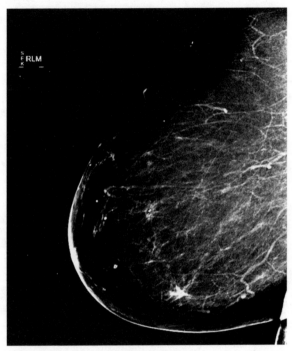

Mammograms use x-rays to image the breast.

Sometimes, a woman finds a new abnormal lump in the breast tissue. Many women have breasts that are naturally lumpy, but if a lump grows or a new lump develops this might warrant a more thorough evaluation. While most breast cancers are not painful, some are and should not be ignored just because they are painful.

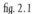

Nurse's Note:

Make your monthly self breast exam a priority. Remember, you may just save your own life.

Occasionally, breast cancer presents as a red, inflamed breast. This condition, also known as **inflammatory breast cancer**, can mimic an infection and can sometimes be difficult for physicians to diagnose. A red, painful breast should always prompt a phone call and visit to a provider for further evaluation.

What Are The Common Causes/Risk Factors Of Breast Cancer?

Many women believe that because they have no family history of cancer they are not at risk for development of breast cancer. In fact, the greatest risk for breast cancer is increasing age in females and **one in eight women over a lifetime** will develop the disease. While men can also develop breast cancer, women get breast cancer 100 times more frequently. Numerous other factors can increase a women's risk for breast cancer. These include family history of breast cancer, having dense breast tissue, being inactive, consuming alcohol, being overweight, delayed childbearing (or not having children), early onset of periods or late menopause, or exposure to hormonal replacement therapies for an extended period of time.

Some things have been shown to **reduce the risk of breast cancer**. These include regular exercise, maintaining a healthy weight, consuming little or no alcohol, and having a first birth at a young age.

About **10% of breast cancers are caused by inherited genetics**, meaning that the risk of developing breast cancer is passed on from generation to generation through an abnormal gene or set of genes. The majority of these cases are caused by a **mutation in the BRCA 1 or BRCA 2 genes**. Generally, the women who develop these cancers have a strong family history of breast cancer, an early age of onset of the cancer (30's to early 40's), and also have an increased risk of ovarian cancer. In these cases, genetic testing can identify the genetic abnormality so that appropriate counseling can be provided to the patient as well as other family members who may be at risk. Some women may opt for prophylactic surgery (removal of the breasts and ovaries) to reduce their risk of breast or ovarian cancer. Others may opt for more intensive surveillance. It should be noted that men can also carry this gene. They may also have an increased risk of breast cancer, an increased risk of prostate cancer, and can pass the genetic abnormality on to daughters and sons.

Unfortunately, there is no way to guarantee that you will not develop breast cancer. However, living a healthy lifestyle, being aware of any changes in your breasts, and having regular mammograms, can help increase the odds that a cancer will be discovered in its earliest stage and have the best prognosis.

Part Three

How Is Breast Cancer Diagnosed?

Breast cancer is discovered in many different ways, but it is always after detection of a change in the breast tissue. Today, most women are diagnosed first by "screening mammography." "Screening" means that there is nothing abnormal to feel, and a test is done to find something different in the tissue. While most differences that appear on mammography are not actually cancer, screening is worthwhile because cancers may be detected before other symptoms are noticed. Cancers are also discovered through self examination, or in conjunction with your doctor. Cancers are also detected because of changes in the appearance of the nipple or skin texture or color.

Breast cancer is **officially diagnosed** when the tissue from a **breast biopsy sample** tests positive. Typically, biopsies will be done if the patient has an abnormal mammogram or if a lump is identified in her breast. If the lump is palpable, the biopsy is sometimes performed by a physician in the office. However, they are usually performed by the radiologist using ultrasound, x-ray, or MRI. The biopsy may eliminate the possibility of cancer. If cancer is detected, then appropriate steps can be taken.

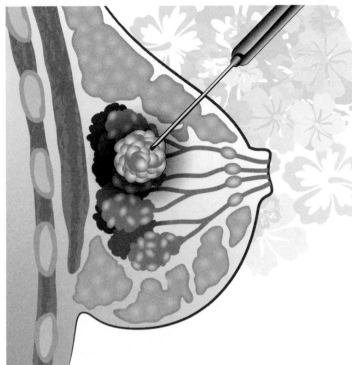

fig. 3.1

Biopsy needles can sample cells from the abnormal area.

Review of imaging

Mammograms are screening tests, which means they are used to detect anything unusual in the breast. If a mammogram is "abnormal" it doesn't automatically mean that there is cancer. It only means that the radiologist sees something different and additional pictures may be needed. The images are compared to previous mammograms if they are available. The findings which may point to cancer are a mass (lump), microcalcifications, or architectural distortion.

You should be able to see your mammograms if you want to. Most mammograms today are done digitally and are easily accessible. It is recommended that you review them with your radiologist or surgeon so that you can see the abnormality and get an idea of its size and what needs to be removed.

Nurse's Note:

When looking up information at the library or on the internet, it is important to know your specific cancer type so that the information is more applicable to you.

If an abnormal mass is detected, further imaging is needed. An ultrasound should be done as a part of the complete work up. If the mass is visible using the ultrasound then a biopsy is recommended. For microcalcifications, if the cluster pattern is suspicious, a stereotactic biopsy is done. An ultrasound is not helpful to better see just microcalcifications. In very special circumstances, usually coordinated with a breast surgeon, a breast MRI may be done before doing a tissue biopsy.

Time For A Biopsy

A core needle biopsy is the preferred method of biopsy and is done with image guidance to take several "cores" or slivers of breast tissue. The pathologist then takes these slivers and examines the cells under a microscope. A core biopsy provides a large sample of tissue which allows more testing on the tissue if a cancer is found. A biopsy can show the type of cancer and other important features.

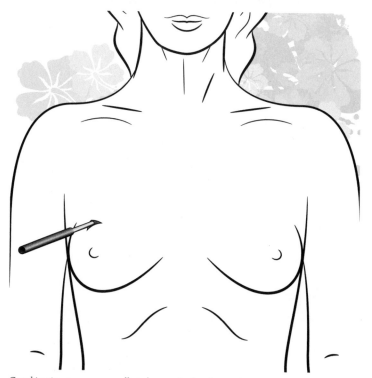

fig. 3.2

Core biopsies remove more cells to be examined under a microscope.

A core biopsy is done with a needle that has a trough to "grab" the tissue and take a core sample. Generally, breast biopsies should be done this way. The needle biopsy is guided by an ultrasound, x-ray, or MRI image of the abnormality to make sure the abnormal area is well sampled. This assures that the abnormal area is not missed by the sampling needle and that the diagnosis of "benign" or "malignant" will have the best chance of being accurate.

Biopsies of a breast abnormality can be done without imaging for very large abnormalities, for obvious findings, or for something that is subtle but is not seen on imaging. Nipple biopsies can also be done by an experienced surgeon without using ultrasound or MRI imaging.

The standard for breast biopsy is image guided core needle biopsy. You can read the American Society of Breast Surgeons Official statement (2006) along with additional references at **www.breastsurgeons.org**. If you have concerns about a needle biopsy, discuss this with your breast surgeon.

Part Four

What Are The Key Factors On A Pathology Report That Help Make Decisions?

Review Of Pathology Report

A medical pathology report can be complicated and, to a patient, seem like it is written in a foreign language. But it can be invaluable in the determination of needed treatments.

The breast is a modified sweat gland, producing milk instead of sweat, full of innumerable ducts running through the breast mound in a variable pattern, branching out and connecting to numerous lobules. The lobules make milk, and the ducts carry milk to the nipple. The breast can be divided into 3 different components. Fat is the largest component, followed by stroma (the fibrous support tissue of the breasts). Ducts and lobules, branching and interacting with the support tissue, make up the smallest component.

Breast cancer is either ductal or lobular in origin. Because the ductal cells outnumber the lobular cells, it is not surprising that ductal cancers are the most common—about 80%. Whether the cancer is ductal or lobular in origin does not make a big difference in treatment.

fig. 4.1

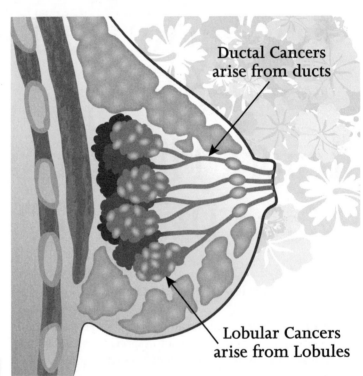

Ductal Cancers arise from ducts

Lobular Cancers arise from Lobules

Different cancer types arise from the ducts and lobules of the breast.

Non-invasive cancers stay within the milk ducts or lobules in the breast. They do not grow into or invade normal tissues within or beyond the breast. These are sometimes called "in-situ" or "pre-invasive cancers". If the cancer has grown beyond where it started, it is called invasive. Most breast cancers are invasive and sometimes spread to other parts of the body through the blood or lymph system.

fig. 4.2

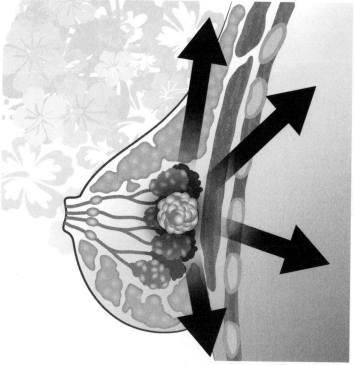

When cancer cells leave the breast, this is called a metastasis.

fig. 4.3

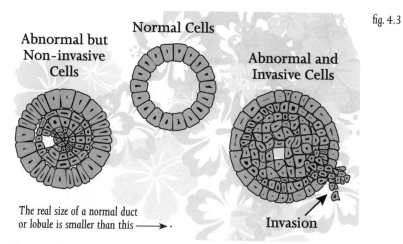

Normal Cells

Abnormal but Non-invasive Cells

Abnormal and Invasive Cells

The real size of a normal duct or lobule is smaller than this ——→ .

Invasion

This is an illustration of a microscopic view of normal ducts and changes leading to abnormal duct cells with invasion.

You May See These Descriptions Of Cancer In Your Pathology Report:

DCIS (Ductal Carcinoma In Situ): This is a cancer that is non-invasive. It stays inside the milk ducts.

LCIS (Lobular Carcinoma In Situ): This is a tumor that is an overgrowth of cells that stay inside the milk-making part of the breast (called lobules). LCIS is not a true cancer. It is a warning sign for an increased risk of developing an invasive cancer in the future, in either breast.

IDC (Invasive or Infiltrating Ductal Carcinoma): This is a cancer that begins in the milk duct but grows into the surrounding normal tissue inside the breast. This is the most common kind of breast cancer.

ILC (Invasive Lobular Carcinoma): This is a cancer that starts inside the milk-making glands (called lobules), but grows into the surrounding normal tissue inside the breast. There are other, less-common types of invasive breast cancer.

A normal duct or lobule is about the size of the period at the end of this sentence. They cannot be seen with the naked eye or felt if touched. This is important to understand. Since ducts or lobules are too small to see, cutting into breast tissue does not give the surgeon much more information about the nature and extent of the cancer than they had going in. Therefore, decisions about whether to have a lumpectomy or mastectomy should be made before surgery, and not during surgery.

Ductal carcinoma in situ (DCIS) means ductal cells have "gone bad." They are cancer and growing out of control, but they cannot "break out" of the ductal lining, which is a thin layer around the ductal cells called a basement membrane. If this membrane is intact, then this cancer is called ductal carcinoma "in situ" by the pathologists. Some people mistake this as "pre-cancer," but it is actually "pre-invasive cancer".

Lobular carcinoma in situ (LCIS) is misnamed and is not actually cancer. It is considered a pre-cancer, or a marker of risk. Removing a spot of LCIS does not remove the risk of cancer.

Biopsy or surgery does not make cancer cells somehow "bust out to become invasive". Only when cells become abnormal and break out of the duct do they become invasive.

Grade is an assessment of how irregular or different the cells are, compared to normal. Grade is not the same thing as "stage," although the two are frequently confused. A low grade tumor is also known as "well-differentiated." It means the cells, while not normal, are usually slower growing and close to normal. Intermediate grade, or "moderately-differentiated," means the cells are between low and high grade. High grade means the cells are markedly different, not normal, and are "poorly differentiated." They tend to be faster growing and generally behave more aggressively.

Tumor size is an important factor when making treatment decisions for breast cancer. Doctors measure cancers in centimeters (cm). The size of the cancer helps to determine its stage.

fig. 4.4

Doctors commonly use centimeters to measure tumors. This is a comparison of millimeters (mm) to centimeters (cm) and inches (in.)

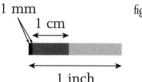

Size is not the only factor. A small cancer can be very fast-growing while a larger cancer can be a slower "gentle giant."

Clinical guesses are made about size by the mammogram and ultrasound and other imaging, as well as by how it feels. The final size is the measurement made by the pathologist after the tissue is removed for examination.

Angiolymphatic invasion, also known as **lymphovascular invasion (or LVI)**, is a characteristic that the pathologist will look for within the tumor specimen. While invasive cells are "out of the duct boundaries," it is a separate risk factor to know that cells are also invading or encircling the blood vessels or lymph channels (LVI). This is a negative feature, since breast cells normally should not have anything to do with invading vessels. The presence of LVI does not mean the cells absolutely traveled out of the breast, and absence of LVI does not mean the cells cannot or did not leave the breast. However, when LVI is present, it raises the risk that the cells have traveled out through the blood or lymph vessels.

fig. 4.5

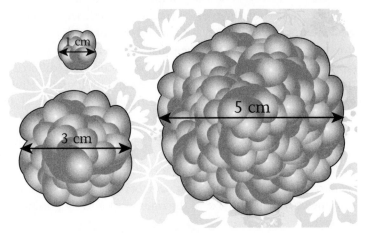

This illustrates sizes of cancer by measured diameters.

Chemical receptors on the surface of breast cancer cells are also studied by the pathologist. All normal breast cells have receptors for estrogen and progesterone, and this means the cells are responsive to any estrogen or progesterone in the bloodstream. It does not matter if a woman is pre- or postmenopausal, or if she is taking estrogen or not, the receptors are always there. If a woman doesn't take any estrogen and she is past menopause, the breast cells normally still have these receptors. They are like antennae on the surface of the cells waiting for estrogen to float by.

As the cells mutate into cancer cells, they may keep, lose, or modify these receptors. The pathologist should automatically test for these receptors on invasive or non-invasive cancers. If the cancer is **estrogen and/or progesterone positive**, it means the cells have kept their normal receptors. This number is usually reported as "positive" with a number, or percentage of the cells, that are positive. If the cells are 0% or very low % positive, they are estrogen and/or progesterone negative, and the cells have lost their normal receptors.

If the cells are significantly estrogen positive, then the cells will be responsive to anti-estrogen medicine to turn them off. The two major types of medications are tamoxifen, a selective estrogen reuptake modulator (SERM), and aromatase inhibitors (AI). There are 3 different AI medications. The selection of which medicine to take and the length of time to take the medication will be made with your medical oncologist. Anti-estrogen therapy is usually given for 5 years (longer duration for some women based on recent date), and, in most cases, is started after completion of surgery, chemotherapy, and radiation (see Part Eight: Radiation Treatment And Breast Cancer, pp. 61–81).

Ki67 is another pathology test to determine how fast the cells are growing. Not every lab does this test. It is given as a percentage and the higher the number, the more aggressive the cells are.

Her2neu is another common receptor the pathologist will test for on invasive cancer cells. This tests positive in about 20% of breast cancers. This receptor is **not** supposed to be there. If it is "**overexpressed**", then it is **Her2neu positive**. Her2neu positive cancers respond better to chemotherapy medicines that attack that receptor. Currently trastuzumab, known by the brand name Herceptin, is the antibody (targeted therapy) to that receptor which is commonly used, but there are other medicines also being studied for this use. Her2neu positive or negative status does not usually change the surgery or radiation plan, but does affect plans for chemotherapy.

Staging

Stage of cancer is an indication of how far the cancer has spread. Non-invasive breast cancer is a stage 0 cancer. Invasive cancer is staged from 1 to 4 (usually using Roman numerals;

Nurse's Note:

Cancer treatments of the future will rely on more genetic testing of cancer cells.

19

I, II, III, IV). Staging takes into account the extent of spread of the disease. The components are how large the primary breast cancer or tumor (T), are there any lymph nodes involved and if so, how many (N), and finally, whether or not the cancer has spread to other places in the body, called a metastasis (M).

Complete staging may not be accomplished until after definitive surgery. At surgery, in addition to removing the tumor and determining its size, lymph nodes are also sampled to see if they are involved. Both size of tumor and lymph node status will determine the stage of disease. Combinations of T, N, and M designations form the stage grouping I – IV.

STAGE GROUPING

• Tumors that are 2 cm or less, without lymph node involvement are Stage I cancers.

• If the tumor is greater than 2 cm and less than 5 cm without lymph node involvement, then the stage is IIA. Tumors 2 cm or less, but with 1-3 lymph nodes involved are also Stage IIA.

• Stage IIB cancers are those tumors greater than 2 cm and less than 5 cm with 1-3 lymph nodes involved, or tumors greater than 5 cm without lymph node involvement.

• Tumors that are larger than 5 cm with any lymph node involvement or tumors that have greater than three lymph nodes involved are designated Stage III.

• Breast cancers that have spread to other organs, such as the liver, bone or brain are designated Stage IV.

Staging is important for several reasons. First, generally the lower the stage, the better the prognosis. Staging also helps determine therapy—whether or not to give chemotherapy, and whether radiation is important after mastectomy. For tumors that are diagnosed in Stage I-III, the goal of therapy at the time of diagnosis is cure. In other words, to prevent the cancer from ever coming back in the breast or in any other part of the body. Unfortunately for patients diagnosed with Stage IV breast cancer, the likelihood of cure is extremely low, and the goal of therapy is palliation. This means giving treatment to control and shrink the tumor and to prolong life and to prevent or control symptoms as long as possible. For many patients with stage IV or metastatic breast cancer this can mean many years. It becomes a disease (like diabetes) that is treated and controlled but not likely "cured".

fig. 4.6

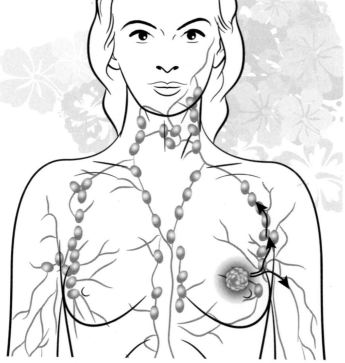

In many cases, the first area of cancer spread from the breast is to the lymph nodes under the arm or under the sternum.

As mentioned, the goal for patients with early (Stage I-III) breast cancer is to cure the disease. Treatment is generally broken into two parts: the local/regional treatment (taking care of the breast tumor and lymph nodes) and the systemic treatment (preventing the cancer from returning in other parts of the body). Many patients wonder why systemic therapy is needed when a small tumor is removed from the breast with no sign of disease in the lymph nodes or in other parts of the body. During the time that the cancer is growing in the breast, one or more cancer cells can escape from the breast, through either the lymph channels, or the blood vessels and settle in another organ. Over time, these cancer cells can grow into larger tumors. The purpose of systemic treatment is to destroy those cells that are potentially hiding, while their size is microscopic. Generally, the greater the stage, the greater the likelihood those cells are out there. However, even small tumors can have the propensity to spread, and so nearly every breast cancer patient is offered some sort of systemic therapy, called Adjuvant (additional) Treatment.

Checklist Of What To Learn About The Radiology And Pathology Reports:

1. What kind of cancer is it?   __Ductal   __Lobular

2. Is it:
   __Invasive   __Non-invasive   __Both invasive
                                                       & non-invasive

3. What is the estimated size? _____

4. What is the grade? (how different are the cells compared to normal)
   __Grade 1   __Grade 2   __Grade 3

5. Is there lymphovascular invasion? (breast cancer cells into the blood
vessels or lymph channels) _____

6. What are the hormone receptors?_____

Estrogen receptors:
   __Positive   __%(0%-100%)   __Negative

Progesterone receptors:
   __Positive   __% (0%-100%)   __Negative

7. What is the Her2neu receptor result?
   __Positive   __Negative   __Borderline

8. What is the best guess about lymph nodes?
   __Positive   __Negative   __Suspicious

Part Five

The Big Picture On Treatment Options: What Factors Make A Difference?

When patients are introduced to the information they need, they are encouraged to "wait for the whole picture." For example, you may feel a lump, or something is found on mammogram. Then you get more mammograms and maybe an ultrasound, then a biopsy, then maybe an MRI, and it can go forward from there. Information rolls out in phases, not just in one single swoop with a single test. It is almost impossible to define the complete treatment plan in one visit. Do not be disappointed if all the answers aren't there in a first visit. Your physicians and care team will help you understand the various pieces to the puzzle that will come together and allow for a treatment plan to be made.

The vast majority of patients with a newly diagnosed breast cancer will be referred first to a breast surgeon. The breast surgeon is usually the coordinator of any additional imaging, work up, and treatment planning. Sometimes the breast surgeon is referred to as the **"captain of the ship,"** and they often set the course for the initial tests and procedures. Breast cancer is a multidisciplinary situation which requires a team of specialists. Most patients will need a breast surgeon, radiologist, medical oncologist, radiation oncologist, and a primary care physician to coordinate your total care. Other specialists who may be added to your team include a plastic surgeon, pathologist, nutritionist, counselor, and physical therapist.

The first consult discussions are filled with new information that you cannot be 100% prepared for. A wide variety of information is usually covered, and you usually will come away from these visits with many handouts and a "to do list." Patients are encouraged to bring a supportive person with them to the first visits because of the volume of information. Some studies suggest that patients only hear about 20% of what is said in these first visits. If you bring someone with you, and they write things down, you can usually retain better than half of what is said. Your support team can be a spouse, family, or friends. They should be someone who is supportive and will be there for you to talk with and bounce your ideas off later.

Nurse's Note:

You will be given a great deal of information during your doctor visits. To keep from being overwhelmed, keep a notebook. Include a list of questions you would like to ask during your visit.

First, Review Everything Else

In general, your doctors will try to review other medical issues first before focusing on the cancer. It is very common for people to forget prior treatments or tests, and not understand how important it is for your treatment team to have a complete picture of your health. If you have had several procedures in the past, or take a number of medicines, it can be helpful to have these details written down before your visits. This way, your doctors will have a complete picture of your health and have adequate time to answer your questions.

Your care team will also try to get a general feel for how you are doing with the cancer diagnosis, how you deal with stress in general, and how they can help. They will try to get an idea of what is important to you, who your support team is going to be, and what else is going on in your life. No woman with breast cancer "has time for it." For some, this seems to hit at the worst time, and others think the timing is better than it could be. Your care team wants to understand the "big picture" and can help put you in contact with support teams that you may not know about. Let them know what is going on in your life, and they will try to help.

Finally!! We Know The Pathology, We've Seen The Imaging, What Do We Do For Treatment?

It can be helpful to draw out on a sheet of paper a personalized review of what steps are needed for treatment.

fig. 5.1

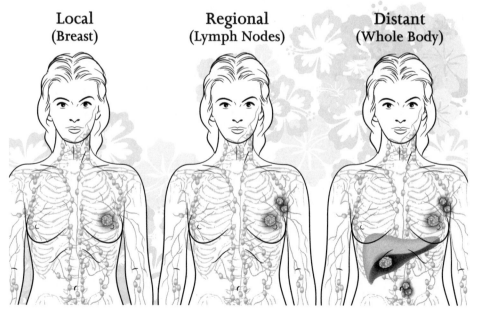

| Local | Regional | Distant |
| (Breast) | (Lymph Nodes) | (Whole Body) |

When making treatment decisions, it is helpful to discuss local, regional and distant treatment approaches separately with your care team.

There typically are 3 basic sections to consider: the **Breast**, the **Lymph Nodes**, and the **Whole Body**. Local (breast), regional (nodes), and systemic (whole body) treatments, while interconnected, are different.

Some patients say, "I want a mastectomy because I don't want chemotherapy". This is an incorrect way of looking at things. The mastectomy may well take care of cancer in the breast, but it doesn't do anything for the cells that may have already left the breast. Other treatments are needed for the rest of the body (such as chemotherapy or hormonal therapy). Chemotherapy, or medicine, can not completely control the cells within the breast on its own, and thus most patients receive a combination of treatments and possibly radiation as well.

What To Do About The Breast

For **the breast**, there are several basic rules. If you work within the rules, then the correct decision can be made even if there are several decisions to choose from.

The first rule is pretty simple—**remove the cancer with a rim of normal tissue**, called a **negative margin**. Basically, you want to get out all the cancer that can be seen microscopically. The pathologist will examine the tissue under the microscope and make a measurement of the margin, or the distance from the edge to the tumor cells.

The second rule is to "**treat**" **the rest of the breast**. In days gone by, everyone just knew a mastectomy was the only choice to "get it all". This was not really true, but other therapies had yet to be designed. When lumpectomy was done, and margins were good, no additional treatment was given. But the recurrence rate was as high as 40%. This was not an acceptable statistic for someone being treated for a cure. Radiation therapy can leave the breast intact and kill the remaining microscopic cancer cells.

Radiation is invisible energy used to treat cancer. Radiation (usually x-ray therapy) is offered because breast cancer cells are inherently radio-sensitive (killed by radiation therapy). Normal cells can recover from the damage caused by radiation, by and large, but the cancer cells cannot. Therefore, the normal cells are more radio-resistant. Now lumpectomy is almost always offered with radiation. It is **very uncommon for radiation and a lumpectomy not to go together**. Physicians who specialize in radiotherapy are called radiation oncologists. If radiation is going to be part of a plan, or even if it is not certain, you will need to see the radiation oncologist at some point to discuss potential benefits and risks for your specific situation.

The third rule is to **check genetics**, or specifically, look for a genetic predisposition to breast cancer, such as BRCA (BRCA is the name of the most common genetic abnormalities that leads to breast cancers in a family). Your care team will go over your family tree with you and look for this risk. By drawing a family tree and discussing who has had cancer, your care team can help you understand if you have an increased risk of this genetic abnormality in your family. Not everyone needs to be tested.

The fourth rule is to **make sure that there is only ONE cancer**. If there are multiple spots of cancer, usually lumpectomy is not advised. There may be some exceptions, but they should be thoroughly reviewed and discussed. Sometimes, this means an MRI or other imaging is done. It depends again upon the specific situation and this will be determined by you with your cancer team.

Lumpectomy Versus Mastectomy?

One common choice for breast treatment is to have a **lumpectomy**, guided by an imaging test to know how much to take out (since the cells can't be seen with the naked eye). As stated earlier, a lumpectomy followed by radiation is one choice. Standard whole breast radiation treatments are the most common and are usually daily for about 15 minutes, Monday through Friday, for about 30-35 treatments over 6-7

Nurse's Note:
Whether you are having a lumpectomy or a mastectomy, it is still surgery. You need to take very good care of yourself while healing. Eat right, take vitamins, and drink plenty of fluids.

weeks. There are some shorter radiation courses. These are discussed in Part Eight: Radiation Treatment And Breast Cancer (pp. 61–81).

fig. 5.2

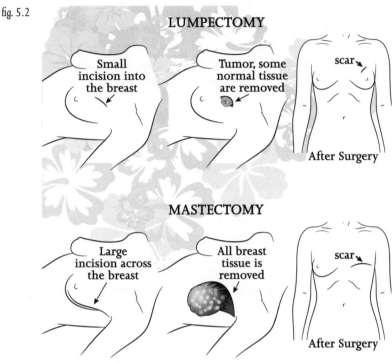

General overview of a lumpectomy versus mastectomy.

The other choice for breast treatment is a **mastectomy**. With a mastectomy, almost all of the breast tissue is removed. A tiny amount remains stuck under the skin. In older days, removing the skin and the chest wall muscle to get every last cell was the goal. That was known as a "radical mastectomy". Usually a skin graft was required because so much was removed down to the ribs. This is almost never done these days. Removing only the breast tissue with a tiny bit left under the skin is called a simple mastectomy. A modified radical mastectomy is the case where the breast and lymph nodes are removed together, with the skin and muscle left intact.

With mastectomy, radiation is not usually needed (with notable exceptions). When radiation after a mastectomy is recommended, it is because there is suspicion that there are breast cancer cells traveling in the skin, the muscles, or lymph nodes. One reason to consider radiation is if there is an invasive tumor greater than 5 cm. If the tumor is this big, it means it has been there for some time and has a much higher chance for cells to be traveling in the skin. The skin will need radiation treatment. The other major reason to give radiation is that lymph nodes are involved with the cancer, thus increasing the chance of "in-transit" cells left behind.

If a mastectomy is done, there are **multiple options for breast reconstruction**. These procedures will be explained to you and coordinated with your breast surgeon and a plastic surgeon. You will need to see a plastic surgeon first to make the full plans and review what choices will work for your situation. If this isn't offered to you, ask why. There may be a good reason. The unavailability of trained plastic surgeons to do these specialized procedures is the most common reason to not be offered reconstruction. However, there are health reasons that can make the procedures less safe. For example, a history of blood clots and blood thinning medicine is a reason not to do cosmetic reconstruction. Smokers are not good candidates for cosmetic reconstruction because smoking inhibits healing. Quitting smoking can help one become a better candidate for reconstruction. Furthermore, if you need radiation after a mastectomy, this can make the cosmetic surgery options more limited and complex. And it is not always known before the initial surgery if radiation is needed after a mastectomy.

What To Do About The Lymph Nodes?

After considering therapies for local treatment of the breast, what to do about the lymph nodes is discussed. Lymph nodes are small structures filled with white blood cells and are connected to the lymph channels that function as filters. They are not perfect filters, but way-stations that monitor the inflow of fluids leaked from capillaries (tiny blood vessels). Lymph nodes do not have anything to do with the sweat glands. Most people would be astounded at how much fluid flows normally every day through the lymph channels, because we don't see the fluid path until something is blocking the path and it doesn't work. The majority of breast fluid flows to the axilla, or armpit. This collection of nodes in the axilla is also the drainage point from the arm and chest wall on the same side. This common pathway accounts for some of the side effects many people have heard about regarding breast cancer (i.e. arm swelling).

The most important predictor of breast cancer risk is the lymph node status, positive (with cancer cells in the nodes) or negative (no cancer cells found in the nodes). To get this information, the nodes are first examined in a physical exam, which is not very accurate in finding small amounts of cancer. The next step is the breast imaging work up, usually with ultrasound. If that is negative, as it usually is, then the nodes most likely to have cancer are taken out, carefully sliced, and examined under the microscope. In past years, the standard was to do an **axillary lymph node dissection**, which meant to take out the nodes at the edge of the breast, called level I and level II nodes. If those nodes were all negative, then it was good news. But since the normal nodes were removed, they could not be replaced, and the information gained (negative nodes) was at a high price. In other words, a patient got all the scar tissue, pain, and risk of arm swelling, without any benefit since no cancer was actually removed. The information was valuable of course, and this was why it was done.

Over time, a standard has evolved called a **Sentinel Node Biopsy**, frequently abbreviated **SLN biopsy**. Sentinel means "guard", and the basic idea is to find the FIRST node or nodes that will drain the breast. The connections of lymph channels leading to the first nodes from the breast is not anatomically the lowest nodes or closest nodes, so it is not something a surgeon will see when they "get in there".

Instead of just guessing, a blue dye is injected into the breast to make a map of which nodes are the first ones. With this map, less nodes will be needed to be taken out to be sure where the cancer might have gone. This is the process of "sentinel node mapping." It is important that the particle be small enough to travel in the tiny lymph channels, and big enough to get trapped in the lymph node filter. Two "dyes" are standard. One is isosulfan blue, a vital dye that is very blue, and the other is technetium-99 labeled radioactive albumin, a natural protein in the body. Today using the radioactive "dye" is the most common, and the blue dye is the back up plan. Talk to your surgeon about specifics since this exact choice has changed often over the last few years, and there are several good protocols specific to each hospital that all work well.

The number of sentinel nodes is variable, ranging from one to several. Wherever the dye goes, that is the pathway that cancer cells might have taken, if they had the ability to travel. The dye will move to the nodes. It is designed to do so. When

Nurse's Note:

Lymphedema is a possible side effect of having lymph nodes removed. If you think you are having any swelling of the arm, tell your nurse and doctor immediately.

fig. 5.3

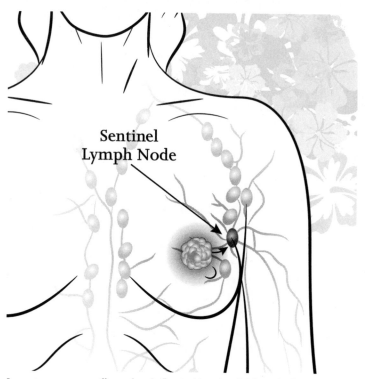

Sentinel
Lymph Node

In most cases, cancer will spread to the "sentinel lymph node" first. This "sentinel node" can be mapped out and removed at the time of surgery.

the dye goes, that does not mean the cancer cells definitely went the same way, it only means that this is the pathway they would have gone. Wherever the dye goes, those are the node(s) that should be removed and tested.

When the sentinel node(s) is identified, and removed, it can be processed by a pathologist to look for cancer cells. While it can be done quickly at the time of surgery, not everyone will necessarily need all their nodes removed. So the nodes are sent out for accurate testing. You and your team will discuss your situation later to determine if more nodes need to be removed. Therefore, when you go home, you won't know whether additional nodes will need to be removed.

This lymph node procedure is usually done at the same time as the breast procedure, either mastectomy or lumpectomy, but there are a few special reasons why it might not. The lymph node procedure is done under general anesthesia. While the breast tissue might be amenable to local anesthesia with sedation, the armpit or axilla is not. There are some nerve blocks that a few physicians use, but even those blocks are not perfect or dependable enough to use just local anesthesia. Ask your surgeon about what to expect, and if you have any special concerns about anesthesia or have a history of a problem with anesthesia, let your surgeon know. Most hospitals allow you to talk to the anesthesiologists ahead of time if there are concerns, but otherwise you will meet them the day of surgery.

What To Do About The Whole Body?

Once you have made the breast and lymph node decisions, and have received those results or predicted results, remember the most important part of you is the rest of you. This is referred to as the **Whole Body**. It isn't the cells in the breast that eventually harm people, it is the cells that leave the breast and establish colonies in other organs. Remember that a centimeter of breast cancer cells, usually too small to feel, contains about a billion cells. A billion cells did not get there over night, and the process of dividing bad cells, one to two, two to four, four to eight, and so forth to get to maybe millions of cells that can be detected takes time. By the time the average 1 cm cancer is found, the bad cells starting the process have been (invisibly) there for several years before detection. It also means that the cells have had plenty of time to travel, if they have the ability, and taking them out of the breast is only part of the treatment. The next determination is how likely it is that the cells invaded the lymph channels or blood stream, traveled to other organs, and set up shop.

This decision on the whole body is a medical oncologist's job. Your breast surgeon is key in coordinating this and determining appropriate timing. Your medical oncologist and breast surgeon will work together to get the treatment plan coordinated.

Your medical oncologist needs information to decide what the offered treatment plan will be. This information helps determine what the risk is that the cancer has spread and if there will be a need for treatment in addition to breast surgery. Unfortunately there is not a tumor marker for all breast cancers. Tumor markers can be measured from the blood to indicate if bad cells are there. The most common tumor marker used in breast cancer patients is CA27-29, but it is only useful in certain circumstance and for select patients.

Since markers will likely not be helpful, other information is needed to make critical treatment decisions. There are **four major factors that your oncologist will consider** in determining the best treatment plan. And if needed, **a fifth factor might be used as a "tie breaker."**

The **first factor is tumor size**. The greater the size the greater the numbers of cells. The more cells there are, the greater the chance that some could mutate and gain the ability to leave the breast and establish a colony somewhere else in the body. In addition, more cells means the tumor has been there longer than one with less cells and therefore has had a greater chance to mutate. Size is not everything, though. Sometimes very small tumors can spread easily and very large tumors may erode through the skin and still not migrate out of the breast. The vast majority of cancers stay in the breast. They do have some potential to spread, however. **The size threshold for considering chemotherapy is about 0.5 to 1.0 cm**. It is not that a centimeter of cancer is going to automatically buy you chemotherapy, but it is a threshold at which chemotherapy should be considered.

The **second factor is lymph node status**. This ranks high on the risk scale. If the nodes are positive (contain cancer cells) the cancer got there by travelling out of the breast. If they came in lymph channels, they might have travelled in the blood stream. Remember, we cannot "see" a million cells in the breast very easily, and therefore it is impossible to see a few cells or even a few hundred cells in the blood stream. If the nodes are negative, that is good, and the risk is less. This does not mean that the cancer cells have not travelled from the breast. It is just less likely.

The **third factor is age and health**. The same treatment offered to a 40 year old might not be appropriate for an 80 year old with the same kind of tumor. The risks for the two are not the same, and the side effects of treatments are not the same. Tumors that look the same under a microscope will not have the same behavior in the 40 year old as they do in the 80 year old. But even if the cells do behave the same, the 40 year old has far more time to have a risk of recurrence than the 80 year old. And that, in turn, may call for a different treatment in the two. Furthermore, a woman's health, including her tolerance level for side effects, needs to be taken into account. Some women are terrified of chemotherapy, for example. In breast cancer treatments there are options to balance risk and side effects. Age and health are taken into consideration in developing the treatment plan.

The **fourth factor is that of "receptor status"**. Namely, estrogen receptor (ER), progesterone receptor (PR) and Her2neu (H2N). If ER is positive, depending on the percentage of positive cells, then **tamoxifen** or **aromatase inhibitors** might be used to treat the cancer. If H2N is positive,

Herceptin (an antibody) might be used with certain chemo-therapies. If ER is negative, then there is no oral medication option, and chemotherapy is more strongly considered. If ER is positive, but there are other bad features like a higher grade or lymphovascular invasion, or large size in a younger woman, then the question might be, "Will anti-estrogen treatments be enough, or will chemotherapy be needed in ad-dition?" In past years, because the risk of missing cancers that had already spread but weren't seen was high, the options was to over-treat with chemotherapy rather than under-treat. Today the balance of the decision – risk of spread versus risk of treatment – is the biggest question in many cancers, in-cluding breast cancer.

There is an extensive research effort to individualize treat-ment, which is why any breast cancer guidebook will never be complete. There are too many factors and there are many studies both past and present that are evolving to guide this decision. Your team will be up to date in these advances and can guide you in making the best decisions for you.

There is a fifth factor, usually described as a tie-breaker. Some small cancers can be lethal and some large cancers are not, so size and nodes are not always the whole story, and some cancers that are ER positive don't respond as well to tamoxifen like they should. If for an ER positive tumor, there are some bad features, then there are new tests that are done on the tumor itself to look for other receptors or genetic fac-tors to predict risk of spread. This technology is evolving, and any trademark tests that are mentioned here might well be out of date and other tests standard a year after this book is printed, so consult with your surgeon and oncologist about the test that might apply to you.

The most common test now is **Oncotype Dx**. This is a test done right on the tumor cells on the slides, to look for other features besides estrogen, progesterone, and Her2neu, to look for genes that might explain how likely a cancer cell is to have travelled. This test was developed from studying cancer cells from the past when the outcome and treatments were known.

If an Oncotype Dx test is done, it is done after surgery, when the size is known (because the cancer was removed and measured,) and the nodes are known. Currently, positive nodes means no tie-breaker is needed, but even that dogma that "everyone knows" is being studied in favor of individualized testing like this.

If the Oncotype score is low, then chemotherapy does not add much benefit, and tamoxifen alone is enough treatment. Everyone in the study of Oncotype took tamoxifen. This is not a test to see if anti-estrogen medicine is needed, it is a test to see if more than that is needed. If the score is intermediate, then more discussion is needed, as some will and some won't need chemotherapy. There is a large clinical trial, called TailoRx, which is done to try and decide what should be recommended when results are in the middle. When the Oncotype Dx is high, the tumor is higher risk to spread, and chemotherapy should be offered.

Oncotype Dx and the other tests like it should not be done for someone who could not have chemotherapy anyway. It should not be done for someone who's tumor features, like size or node status, are not reasons enough to give chemotherapy. It should really be saved as a "tie-breaker" to decide if the cancer is favorable enough to not need chemotherapy.

If you need chemotherapy, it is common to need a port. A port is a small reservoir that is connected to a long IV tube placed into a large vein such as the internal jugular or one of the arm veins. Also, there usually has to be some extra heart tests, such as an echocardiogram or MUGA scan. Blood work is usually done, but the blood work is not to tell us about the cancer as much as to make sure that the rest of the body is doing okay.

Hormonal Therapy Questions

For pre menopausal women, studies have been done to see if the timing of a menstrual cycle affects the outcome of treatment. Studies are conflicting, and most experts do not think

fig. 5.4

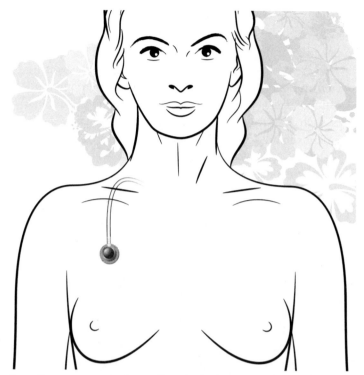

Chemotherapy ports are placed surgically under the skin. This greatly simplifies chemotherapy treatment and other procedures such as blood draws and IVs.

that waiting for a part of a cycle to happen is helpful, but that surgery, chemotherapy and radiation should proceed regardless. It is normal to have regular cycles become irregular with stress of any surgery.

For pre-menopausal women on oral contraception, this should be discontinued as soon as feasible. With cycle irregularities, expect the unexpected, and plan for appropriate barrier contraception such as condoms for sexual activity. This is a good time to discuss options with your breast surgeon and medical oncologist.

For pre-menopausal women, the chances of conceiving after most breast cancer treatments are lower. If you want to preserve options of fertility, you need to talk to your surgeon very soon after diagnosis.

For women peri- or post- menopausal, hormone replacement should not be taken. If you are on hormones, you need to talk to your doctors about how to come off. There is no case where with a new breast cancer diagnosis that hormones are recommended. This includes typical estrogen only prescriptions such as premarin or estrace. It includes combinations such as estrogen with progesterone, and even testosterone. This includes shots, pills, patches, troches, and creams. This also includes bio-identical hormones. All hormones stimulate the breast tissue when your treating doctors want to turn off the breast tissue. Even hormone negative breast cancers are an indication for stopping hormones. Very seldom should hormone treatments be offered, but the details of the possible exceptions can be reviewed with your doctors.

Loss of hormones affects women differently. If you have symptoms, talk it over with your doctor because treatment options are very individual. Vaginal dryness and difficulty with urination, and other symptoms in that area are treated differently than hot flashes and night sweats. There are non-hormonal treatments to help manage some of those symptoms.

What Is The Difference Between Metastatic And Non-Metastatic Cancer? What Is A Metastasis And Is Surgery An Option For Metastatic Disease?

A metastasis is a breast cancer cell that has left the breast and gone to another site in the body. If a breast cancer is growing in the bone, it is not "bone cancer" but breast cancer metastatic to the bone.

There is no such thing as an "encapsulated" breast cancer. There is no breast "capsule" to contain the cells. With non-invasive cancer, or ductal carcinoma in situ, the breast cancer cells do not have access to the lymph channels or blood vessels to travel and therefore are not expected to cause a metastasis. The trouble in saying this is zero risk of spread is the difficulty in proving that there is no invasive component at all.

Nurse's Note:
Remember your notebook! Your doctor will give you information you will want to write down.

40

With invasive cancer, the cells may or may not have the capacity to separate from their counterparts, enter the blood stream or lymph vessels, and travel to other locations. This is a process that is under ongoing study, and individual to each tumor.

There are some theories on how breast cancer spreads which suggest that tumor cells "recirculate" and return to the breast and re-spread. It is known that patients who have had primary tumor resection, such as a lumpectomy or mastectomy, and then were discovered to already have metastasis, did better in survival compared to women who were found to have metastasis and did not have surgery because it was thought to be a useless control. This is a complex decision, but there is an indication in favor of removal of the breast cancer in the breast area even when there is known spread outside of the breast.

Summary Of What You Should Know By The End Of Your First Consults:

• You should have an understanding of the type of tumor and about how big it is thought to be.

• You should have a plan as to whether additional imaging is needed.

• You should have an understanding about some of the pathology information like grade and receptors.

• You should have an idea of the two basic choices for breast management – lumpectomy and radiation versus mastectomy, and how this is usually separate from the whole body treatment. And you should have an idea of long term results from both of these approaches.

• If a mastectomy is planned, you should have an idea of reconstruction options and timing.

• You should understand your plan for lymph node assessment, such as sentinel node biopsy and timing.

• You should have an idea of how likely chemotherapy is going to be, and how to gather that info to decide (size, node status, age/health, receptor status, and tie-breaker).

• You should have a plan for when you need to see the medical oncologist – before surgery or after.

• If you have a larger tumor, or Her2neu positive tumor, or positive nodes you may have a reason to do chemotherapy before surgery. This is called neoadjuvant chemotherapy, and you would see the medical oncologist to formulate a plan.

• You should know about genetic information and whether you need BRCA testing and how to use it. And whether you need to see a genetics counselor for additional testing.

• You should take stock of your feelings, and know who to turn to for support. There is no single normal way to take all this in.

• You should have an idea of how to incorporate other health issues and changes to your life, and perhaps seek nutritional counseling.

• You should have a plan for counseling with and using the needed team members: breast surgeon, medical oncologist, radiation oncologist, plastic surgeon, counseling, radiologist, physical therapist.

Part Six

What Are My Surgical Options And How Do I Decide?

Surgeons are responsible for removing the tumor, and deciding the best way to do this involves knowing the imaging as well as the exam of the breast. Since surgery is not the only treatment for most breast cancer, surgeons should be the guide for breast cancer patients in the whole treatment of breast cancer.

What Types Of Surgery Are There?

First there needs to be an outline of the treatment plans, separating the decisions on breast surgery from the decisions regarding lymph node surgery and "whole body" treatments. There are a few rules to help make these decisions.

The first "rule" is to remove all the cancer with a rim of normal tissue, or negative margins. This sounds simple, but is a good starting point to decide surgery.

43

If this was all that was needed, mastectomy would have worked centuries ago and no other treatment needed to be invented. Recurrence after lumpectomy alone can be as high as 40%. Breast cancer cells can have local "satellites" in the breast that may not be seen on imaging or felt and lead to recurrence in the breast. Those satellites need to be "treated" by adding radiation after lumpectomy or with mastectomy. Post mastectomy radiation is usually not needed, unless there are risk factors that the cancer cells might be already in the skin, muscle, or lymph nodes. Large tumor size, usually greater than 5 cm, and positive nodes, are generally reasons for this.

The third "rule" is to show that there is only one tumor. If the tissue is very dense and difficult to examine with mammogram, or was found as a lump that isn't visible on mammogram, then breast magnetic resonance imaging (MRI) or positron emmission mammography (PEM) is needed to rule out multiple spots of cancer. This is a complex decision that should be reviewed with your surgeon.

The fourth "rule" is to carefully review and decide that there is not a genetic predisposition to breast cancer. BRCA testing and genetic counseling should be considered and ruled out as a component before considering lumpectomy.

A lumpectomy is a surgery to remove the tumor with a rim of normal tissue. A mastectomy is the removal of virtually all of the breast tissue. A lumpectomy alone is very seldom the treatment. Radiation is a key component and is recommended to follow lumpectomy.

The breast surgeon will make a decision based on imaging and exam as to how much tissue should be removed to get a good margin, or a rim of normal tissue around the tumor. Sometimes this gives a bad "tumor to breast ratio" where removing the area leaves an unacceptable cosmetic defect.

A mastectomy may be needed when the volume of tissue to be removed is so high that the result is unacceptably deformed. Also, tumors that are multiple and therefore making lots of satellites are almost never successfully treated with lumpectomy. If radiation cannot be offered, such as in some cases of connective tissue disorder or a history of prior radiation, then mastectomy is needed.

Strong family history of breast cancer, positive testing for a mutation in the BRCA genes or other breast cancer genes, and personal history of atypical hyperplasia are other reasons to consider mastectomy more for prevention of the next risk of cancer than for treatment of the current cancer.

Survival should not be determined by the local treatment of the breast, as long as the rules are considered. Women who have a lumpectomy and radiation should have comparable survival to women who have a mastectomy for the same tumor factors. Recurrence rates may be different, but survival should be the same. If a woman is treated with lumpectomy and radiation, and it recurs or comes back in the breast, then mastectomy is almost always needed to remove it because more radiation is not typically possible.

Reconstruction options can be considered at the same time as mastectomy in appropriate situations.

How Is A Plastic Surgeon Involved For Reconstruction And Who Is A Good Candidate?

The breast surgeon should be the guide in breast treatment options. If a mastectomy is needed for treatment, reconstruction options should be discussed. Coordination between the plastic surgeon and the breast surgeon is a key factor to good treatment.

Availability of **plastic surgeons skilled in breast reconstruction** is a limiting factor. Seek out a plastic surgeon through your breast surgeon or through reputable organizations such as **plasticsurgery.org**, the website for American Board Certified Plastic Surgeons.

There are two basic types of reconstruction which can be

immediate or delayed. Immediate means that a breast is removed and a reconstruction is done at the same time as removal. Delayed means that a breast is removed and the area healed, and a reconstruction is done at any point later. To be eligible for reconstruction, a woman needs to be healthy enough for the additional surgery.

The **most common type of reconstruction is to use implants, silicone or saline**, to make a breast mound. There are some variations in how to make a breast mound with artificial skin or latissimus flaps to cover the implant. The other way to make a breast mound is to use your own tissue. The most common way to do this is to use the lower abdominal fat, in a procedure called a transverse rectus abdominal musculocutaneous flap transfer, also commonly known as a TRAM. There are some variations in how this is done as well, with a "free TRAM" or a DIEP (deep inferior epigastric perforator) flap.

fig. 6.1

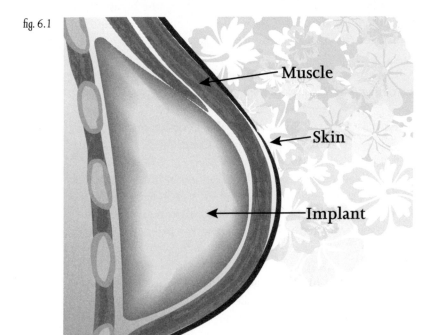

Muscle

Skin

Implant

A breast implant is, in most cases, inserted below the skin and muscle and over the chest wall.

There are some contraindications to reconstruction surgery. Other than overall health for having any surgery, reconstruction is not done in smokers or those who use any nicotine. Severe obesity and history of blood clots are relatively strong reasons not to do reconstruction. If a breast cancer patient needs radiation after mastectomy, the issue is complicated.

What Technologies Are Available In This Modern Era To Improve Surgery And Healing?

Surgery techniques have improved gradually over the years so that there is no single technique in the last decade to point to as a definite change. Techniques with electrocautery to minimize trauma to the tissue have improved. Better understanding of anesthesia techniques on cancer treatment, and improvements in anesthesia have made treatment easier to tolerate and recover from than in prior decades. In addition, a sentinel lymph node biopsy is a less extensive surgery to evaluate the lymph node status and reduces complications when compared to a traditional lymph node dissection.

How Do You Prepare Patients For Surgery (Tests)?

There are published guidelines for pre-surgical testing depending on age. For evaluation of a newly diagnosed breast cancer, not just for surgery but for treatment, complete blood counts and electrolytes and liver function tests should be done. Other medical problems have to be optimized, such as diabetes and hypertension, for surgery or treatment. EKG is needed, depending on age and heart history. Chest x-ray is considered a standard to evaluate for breast cancer metastasis, but the yield on this test is low. It is a pretty simple, less expensive test, which is still usually done, especially to get a baseline exam for the lungs and ribs before treatment. In women still menstruating without tubal ligation, pregnancy test is standard.

Most pre-surgery preparation is education on what to expect for anesthesia and surgical recovery, return to activity, and anticipation of results.

Nurse's Note:
Any surgical procedure has the chance for infection. Signs may be fever, redness, pain, swelling, and/ or warmth of the area. Let your nurse know if you experience any of these symptoms.

What Will Happen On The Day Of Surgery?

The activity on the day of surgery will of course depend on the surgery planned. If a lumpectomy is planned, then a way to localize the tumor is needed. Typically, a localizing wire may be placed in the breast guided by ultrasound or mammogram or MRI, depending on the way the tumor is best viewed. This is done with local anesthesia and is usually much easier on a person than the biopsy. If you are experiencing considerable stress, oral anti-anxiety medication may be used before the procedure. Letting your surgeon know of your anxiety before the procedure will make it easier to coordinate.

If a mastectomy is planned, then there is no need for a localizing wire technique. A patient would be marked pre-op with a marker on the skin to affirm the correct procedure.

If you are having mastectomy with reconstruction, the plastic surgeon may mark you even more extensively preoperatively and even take pictures to document the "before" pictures for intraoperative guidance to rebuild. Some surgeons might do this in the day(s) before the surgery and some might do it the same day.

For surgery, there is a **wide variety of anesthesia techniques** but there is a common need for some type of general anesthesia. If you have ever had issues with anesthesia, let your surgeon know so that appropriate preparation and alternatives are reviewed. You should ask if there are blocks available, injections of local anesthesia to lessen post operative pain. Talk to your surgeon about your expectations for pain management, so that you are not having this discussion when you are already in pain.

In many cases, breast cancer cells will spread first to lymph nodes located in the axilla, or armpit area (adjacent to the affected breast). However, in breast cancers close to the center of the chest (near the sternum), cancer cells can also spread to lymph nodes inside the chest (under the sternum).

A sentinel lymph node is by definition the first regional lymph node (or nodes) to which cancer cells spread from the original primary tumor. In some cases, there can be more than one sentinel lymph node. In fact, the national average by some studies for the number of sentinel lymph nodes is 3. When cancers spread to lymph nodes, this is a key factor (or marker of increased risk) that signals to doctors that the cancer cells could also be spreading through the bloodstream to other parts of the body (microscopic cancer seedlings). Of course the entire bloodstream cannot be tested, so physicians will utilize the lymph nodes to give a statistical risk assessment of the cancers spread to other parts of the body.

What Is A Sentinel Lymph Node Biopsy?

A sentinel lymph node biopsy (SLNB) is a surgical procedure during which the sentinel lymph node (or nodes) is identified, surgically removed, and examined by pathology to determine whether cancer cells have spread to the lymph node.

A "negative SLNB result" means that the pathologist did not find cancer in the lymph node(s). A "positive SLNB result" indicates that cancer is present in the sentinel lymph node. This information can help a doctor determine the stage of the cancer and develop an optimal treatment plan.

What Happens During An SLNB?

A surgeon injects a radioactive substance, a blue dye, or both near the breast tumor to find the position of the sentinel lymph node. The surgeon then utilizes a machine that detects radioactivity to locate the sentinel node or looks for lymph nodes that have been stained with the blue dye.

The sentinel node is then analyzed under a microscope for the presence of cancer cells by a pathologist. If cancer cells are found, the surgeon may than remove additional lymph nodes, either during the same biopsy procedure or during a follow-up surgical procedure.

What Are The Potential Benefits Of SLNB?

In addition to helping your care team stage cancers, SLNB allows some patients to avoid more extensive lymph node surgery. Removing additional nearby lymph nodes to look for cancer cells may not be necessary if the sentinel lymph node is negative for cancer. All lymph node surgery can have side effects, and many of these effects may be reduced or avoided with a SLNB.

Most lumpectomies are done as outpatients. It may take most of the day, but seldom do patients spend the night in the hospital unless there is another issue. Most mastectomy patients stay overnight, but some go home later the same day. This gives patients more time to adjust to the drains necessary after mastectomy, but seldom used with lumpectomy and sentinel node biopsy. If reconstruction is done, the time may be longer, depending on if one breast or both are done, and what the type of reconstruction is. It is very uncommon to stay in the hospital more than 23 hours after a mastectomy.

What Are The Common Problems That Can Occur After Surgery And How Are They Treated?

The most common problem after breast surgery is **infection**. The breast is considered a "clean" area compared to other sites, like mouth surgery or intestinal surgery, but there are germs present that cannot be completely eliminated. The risk of an infection after surgery is estimated at a few percent up to 20-30% of cases, depending on how the infection is defined. Redness without abscess (infected tissue pocket) that might be treated with antibiotics is more common. Abscesses with pus that might need additional drainage or surgery is much less common. Redness that is new, generally begins day 5-7 after surgery.

A much less common problem is **bleeding after surgery**. Increased swelling may occur usually soon after surgery, maybe as early as when you are in the recovery room or the first day after surgery. Some swelling is expected, and it can be

Nurse's Note: Your nurse will ask you to rate your pain on a scale of 1-10, with 1 being the least amount of pain and 10 being the worst, so she can help the doctor adjust pain medicines to help keep you comfortable.

difficult to tell, so if there is a question, it needs to be seen by your surgeon. The treatment is usually a washout of the area in surgery to identify and stop the bleeding, and to remove the blood to prevent thick scar tissue. The earlier this is done the more successful it is. It is very rare to need a transfusion due to bleeding and it is not necessary to donate blood ahead of time for breast surgery.

Longer term effects are **changes in sensation and possibly pain**. No matter how simple, when the breast tissue is removed with lumpectomy or mastectomy, nerves to the breast and the chest wall area can be disrupted. They may be numb or "irritated" or painful for an unpredictable time. Some chronic discomfort may be present to a degree indefinitely, although in general, most pain does improve and is manageable. Sometimes, the response is hard to predict.

A mastectomy is not usually more painful than a lumpectomy. The breast nerves going through the breast are removed, and they are not there to report pain to the brain, thus after mastectomy, numbness is more common than pain. Even reconstruction is not sensate, or in other words, the reconstructed breast does not "feel normal".

After any surgery, it is possible to have problems with wound healing. The tissue may collect more edema or fluid, stretching the incision and preventing healing. Appropriate support and minimization of trauma to the area should be discussed pre-operatively. In general for patients who have a lumpectomy, there should be no "bouncing or banging". Avoid letting the breast tissue bounce without support, and avoid reaching across the chest and "banging" into the breast. Wearing a bra usually provides good support to help prevent the trauma.

With a mastectomy, the skin over the breast is closed over the muscle. The blood supply to the skin used to be through the breast, and now the skin has to adapt to less supply through the thin skin. **Smoking, obesity, prior scar tissue, and relative malnutrition are factors that affect healing**

negatively. Specifics on drain care and the role of drains should be reviewed with your surgeon. In general, the recently removed tissue leaves 2 surfaces that weep normal body fluid similar to plasma. If this fluid is not actively removed it will collect and prevent the skin and muscle from opposing and healing together. Surgical drains which pull fluid out by suction into a bulb are standard. They are designed to pull the fluid out and keep it from returning back into you while healing.

The Potential Side Effects Of Lymph Node Surgery Include The Following:

• *Lymphadema*, or nearby tissue swelling. During SLNB or more extensive lymph node surgery, the regional lymph vessels leading to and from the sentinel node (or group of nodes) are cut. This disruption may lead to an abnormal back-up of lymph fluid. In addition to swelling, women with lymphedema may experience pain or discomfort in the affected tissues (the arm for example), and the overlying skin may become tight or thickened. In addition, there is an increased risk of infection in the affected area or arm.

• *Seroma*, or the buildup of lymph fluid within the surgical cavity.

• *Numbness*, tingling, or pain sensation at the site of the surgery.

• *Difficulty moving* the affected body part.

• *Short term discoloration of the skin* from the dye utilized for the SLNB.

Part Seven

What Is Chemotherapy And What Will I Experience With Chemotherapy?

Chemotherapy is a type of cancer treatment taken by mouth or put into the blood stream through an IV that treats your whole body for cancer. A medical oncologist will determine if chemotherapy is needed or recommended in your situation.

Chemotherapy can, in some cases, be given before surgery (Neoadjuvant Chemotherapy). Your team of care providers will review the specifics of your situation to determine the optimal sequence of therapies.

For Breast Cancer, There Are Three General Categories Of Treatment.

Nurse's Note:

Your Physician may not give you chemo if your blood counts are too low. This is for your safety.

Not all therapies are appropriate for every patient. 1) For patients with tumors that are positive for the estrogen receptor and/or the progesterone receptor, hormonal therapy is an important part of treatment. Generally this is given orally, and for a minimum of five years. 2) Patients who have tumors which have Her2neu receptors (H2N) are eligible for Her-2neu directed therapies such as **trastuzumab** (Herceptin). Generally this is given in conjunction with chemotherapy. 3) The third type of treatment is chemotherapy. Chemotherapy is given intravenously, usually for a period of about 4-6 months, after surgery. Sometimes chemotherapy is offered prior to surgery to shrink the tumor and give more options for surgical resection. Chemotherapy is often used in tumors that are larger, node positive, or estrogen and progesterone receptor negative. Special genetic testing is now available for tumors to help determine the risk of recurrence and the benefit of chemotherapy. Two such tests are Oncotype Dx and Mammoprint.

Nurse's Note:

Most facilities offer a chemo class prior to you starting therapy. This is a great way to learn about the drug you will be given and specific side effects it may have.

What Are The Common Chemotherapy Treatments For Breast Cancer?

The most common chemotherapy agents used in breast cancer include Adriamycin, Cytoxan, Taxol, and Taxotere. These medications are administered every 1-3 weeks depending on the precise regimen being used.

If your doctor recommends chemotherapy, certain side effects are common. These include fatigue, hair loss, nausea, increased risk of infection, and anemia. Generally these side effects are temporary and resolve within a few weeks to months before the end of chemotherapy. Chemotherapy can have delayed effects as well. These include damage to the heart muscle, or cardiomyopathy, damage to the nerves resulting in peripheral neuropathy, and the increased risk of secondary blood cancers such as leukemia, and myelodysplasia. It is important to speak with your doctor regarding the

Nurse's Note:

There are many home care companies that can be supportive during times of need.

toxicities as well as the benefits of chemotherapy to determine if it is the right treatment for your disease.

fig. 7.1

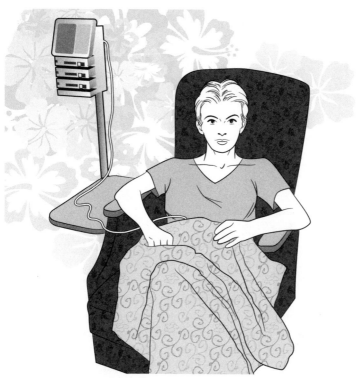

During IV Chemotherapy, you will be monitored while relaxing in a comfortable chair for a couple of hours with the chemotherapy being infused into your bloodstream.

Often when chemotherapy is administered, a port is placed in the arm or chest. This makes it safer and simpler to give the chemotherapy agents, which can be quite damaging to peripheral veins (see fig. 5.4 pg. 39). The port is usually placed while in the operating room under sedation and can be easily removed at the conclusion of chemotherapy. Typically, on a chemotherapy day, you will have a visit with the provider, as well as lab work to make sure that is it safe to proceed with chemotherapy. Chemotherapy treatments are preceded by anti-nausea medications either given by mouth or intravenously. The actual administration of the chemotherapy drugs takes a few hours, and is usually performed in an outpatient setting.

Nurse's Note:

Your nurse can help you manage side effects of therapy. Let your nurse or doctor know about any changes in the way you are feeling.

fig. 7.2

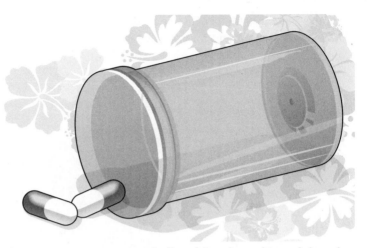

There are many new ways to treat side effects of chemotherapy that greatly lessen the degree of side effects experienced.

Often patients feel fairly well for the first 24-48 hours, and then the symptoms worsen for a few days. The symptoms experienced with chemotherapy can vary greatly from patient to patient, even when the same medications are used. Often fatigue is cumulative, but if your symptoms are well managed with the first round of chemotherapy, generally the next rounds will go well also. If you do develop symptoms, such as severe nausea, rash, or bowel problems, it is important to communicate with your doctor so that these issues can be addressed early. If hair loss is expected from chemotherapy, it generally occurs 2-3 weeks after the first chemotherapy treatment is given, and stays out until chemotherapy is complete.

What Are The Common Hormonal Therapies For Breast Cancer?

Hormonal therapies are used for breast cancers which are positive for estrogen and/or progesterone receptor. These treatments include the medication tamoxifen, or a group of drugs called aromatase inhibitors. Side effects include exacerbation of menopausal symptoms such as hot flashes and sleep disturbances. Tamoxifen, primarily used for premenopausal women, can increase the risk of uterine cancer and the risk of blood clot. It has also been shown to increase the risk of cataracts. Aromatase inhibitors can cause osteoporosis and increase the risk of bone fractures. They also commonly cause joint and muscle aches and pains. These medications are usually prescribed for five years. Recent studies however, have shown the value of taking these medications for longer periods of time and suggest that doing so may decrease the risk of relapse of breast cancer 10-20 years after diagnosis.

Medications can help lessen the side effects of these drugs. A common anti-depressant, venlafaxine, has been shown to reduce hot flashes. Acupuncture, exercise and a healthy diet may also help in reducing some of the more common symptoms. For patients on an aromatase inhibitor, exercise can help preserve bone density, and medications are also available to help prevent bone loss. Calcium and Vitamin D intake are also important.

Many patients experience anxiety and depression at some point during their breast cancer treatment. Mental health professionals, support groups, and on-line chat groups can be very helpful during this time. It is also important to acknowledge the impact of the diagnosis and treatment on family members of the patient. Support for them can often relieve the stress on the patient as well.

Nurse's Note:
Mental health professionals are not just available for the patient. They can help families gain coping skills as well.

What Other Therapies Are Available For The Treatment Of Metastatic Breast Cancer?

Women with advanced breast cancer at diagnosis, as well as those who have a recurrence of breast cancer, have many treatment options available. Local recurrence refers to breast cancers that come back in the same breast as the original cancer, or on the chest wall after mastectomy. Often these tumors can be removed surgically, or a mastectomy can be performed if a patient originally had a lumpectomy. Additional treatment, such as chemotherapy and/or radiation therapy is often also offered, depending on the circumstances.

For women with stage IV or metastatic cancer, control of disease and symptoms remains the most important goal of therapy. Depending on the characteristics of the breast cancer, many treatment options are available and include chemotherapy, hormonal therapy, and for appropriate patients, Her2neu directed therapy. Instead of a prescribed number of treatments or length of treatment, therapy is very individualized, and disease response and patient tolerance are the most important considerations. These treatments can go on for years. Response to therapy can be measured using imaging such as CT scans, or MRI scans. Blood tests for tumor markers may also be appropriate for certain patients. Radiation therapy may also be utilized for brain metastases, symptomatic bone metastases, and newer techniques may be used for limited lung or liver metastases (SBRT or stereotactic body radiotherapy—see Part Eight: Radiation Treatment And Breast Cancer, pp. 61–81). In addition, radiation may be helpful for enlarged lymph nodes that may be causing symptoms. Patients with bone metastases should receive medication to strengthen bones and prevent bone fractures.

Breast Cancer Follow Up

Women with a history of breast cancer require lifelong follow up. Generally, patients are seen for a cancer directed history and physical every 3-4 months for the first three years after diagnosis, every six months during year 4 and 5, and annually after. Women should have annual mammograms to evaluate any remaining breast tissue. In addition, women on tamoxifen should have annual pelvic exams. No routine imaging studies are recommended other than mammograms. However, symptom directed imaging should be performed if warranted. An example of this would be performing a bone scan or hip x-ray if a patient presented with persistent hip pain. Although many breast cancer recurrences can present during the first five years after diagnosis, we now know that delayed breast cancer recurrences are not uncommon. These recurrences can present years and even decades after the initial diagnosis. Current research involves trying to identify genetic markers that may indicate those women at risk for late recurrences. Perhaps those women would be appropriate candidates for extended hormonal treatment.

Lifestyle choices and habits can have a significant impact on breast cancer recurrence and survival. Much of this research has emerged in the last decade. Alcohol consumption is a risk factor for both new breast cancer as well as breast cancer recurrence. The more alcohol consumed on a regular basis, the greater the risk, with the least risk associated with abstinence.

Exercise has also been shown to greatly reduce the risk of breast cancer recurrence and risk of death from breast cancer. Most studies indicate that exercising between 30 and 45 minutes daily, is adequate. Relevant exercise includes walking, swimming and bike riding at a moderate pace. Women who have not been active prior to diagnosis can also benefit, and women of all body types will benefit from exercise.

Although specific dietary interventions have not been shown to significantly alter breast cancer recurrence risk, some recommendations can be made. One study has shown that a low fat diet may reduce the risk of recurrence in patients with estrogen receptor negative breast cancer. Other studies have shown that even modest weight loss can improve risk of recurrence, particularly in postmenopausal women.

Physical therapy to restore range of motion and to treat lymphedema can be very beneficial. Many women going through breast cancer treatment also benefit from complimentary therapy. This can include acupuncture, support groups, and massage. These treatments can help manage nausea, fatigue, depression and pain.

Part Eight

Radiation Treatment And Breast Cancer

What Is Radiation Therapy? How Does It Work?

Radiation therapy uses energy rays or radioactive particles to eradicate cancer cells from healthy body tissues.

Radiation affects cancer cells by interacting with our DNA. DNA is located in every cell in our bodies and acts like a little instruction manual. It is essential for keeping our tissues working normally. Because DNA is so important, normal cells have highly sophisticated machinery for repairing it. When DNA is damaged, normal cells stop and repair it. If the damage is too extensive to repair, the normal cell self-destructs. This prevents the damaged DNA from being passed on to future cells. When cells become cancerous, they lose the ability to repair damaged DNA. This allows cancer cells to accumulate mutations and spread. Cancer cells are more sensitive to radiation therapy (damaged and killed more easily) than healthy cells.

Radiation therapy is typically given over many small doses or fractions. Each dose causes a small amount of DNA dam-

fig. 8.1

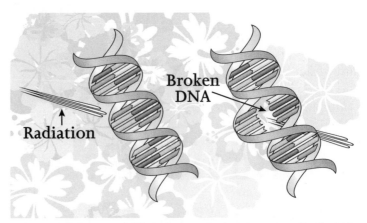

Radiation works by causing breaks in the DNA strands within cancer cells. This leads to cancer cell death.

age. Cells in healthy normal tissues will stop and repair this damage. But cancer cells continue trying to divide and grow without repairing the damaged DNA. When a cancer cell whose DNA has been damaged by radiation tries to divide, it dies. Other mechanisms also help radiation kill cancer cells while sparing normal tissues. This is especially important in breast cancer treatment because cancer cells are often interspersed throughout healthy tissues.

There are several ways of producing radiation. Radiation can come from radioactive materials, or it can come from a specialized machine that generates a radiation beam. Breast radiation therapy is most often done with **external beam radiation**. In external beam radiation, high energy x-rays are produced by a machine called a **linear accelerator**. The x-rays used for radiation treatment are similar to those used for a chest x-ray or CT scans but using higher energy. Like regular x-rays, you cannot see or feel the beam while it is on. As soon as the machine is turned off, the radiation stops.

Radiation can also be delivered from a small radioactive source placed inside the body. This is called **brachytherapy**. The radioactive source is then removed from the patient after treatment. Regardless of how the radiation is produced, all forms of radiation have identical effects on our cells.

Nurse's Note:

Depending upon the goals of treatment, radiation courses can range from 1–7 weeks.

Radiation therapy has similarities to both surgery and chemotherapy. Like surgery, radiation therapy is a local form of treatment. It targets areas at high risk for cancer, or tumors that cannot safely be removed with surgery. Like chemotherapy, radiation can kill microscopic cancer cells without destroying or removing healthy tissues. But since radiation can be focused on specific areas, it is more effective than chemotherapy at controlling cancer in a specific body region.

When Is Radiation Used For Breast Cancer?

Radiation can be used after lumpectomy or mastectomy to prevent cancer from returning. When radiation is given after surgery, it is referred to as **curative** treatment. The goal of therapy in this situation is to kill microscopic cancer cells that remain. If cancer has spread to another organ, radiation treatment is referred to as **palliative**. The goal of palliative radiation is to relieve symptoms caused by a tumor.

What Are Radiation Options Following Lumpectomy?

Over the last 40 years, thousands of women have been treated in clinical trials comparing lumpectomy to mastectomy. These studies demonstrated that after lumpectomy, the risk of cancer recurring within the breast is relatively high if radiation is not given; up to 40%. In contrast, women who receive radiation after lumpectomy have the same chance of cure as women undergoing mastectomy. In other words, adding radiation therapy makes lumpectomy as effective as mastectomy. For this reason, lumpectomy followed by radiation is the standard treatment for women with early stage breast cancer.

Nurse's Note:

It is important that you keep all of your appointments for radiation treatment for optimal results. If you miss a session, it may be added to the end of treatment.

After lumpectomy, radiation reduces the risk of cancer recurrence in the breast by about 70%. But in select cases, the risk of recurrence after surgery alone may already be very low (<10% chance). This is often the case after lumpectomy for some women with small amounts of DCIS as well as in women over 70 who have small, hormone receptor positive cancers. While radiation always decreases the likelihood that the cancer will return, some patients at low risk for recurrence may choose to omit radiation.

Radiation therapy is directed at the areas that are most likely to have residual cancer. After a lumpectomy, the area at highest risk for recurrence of cancer is the tumor bed (lumpectomy cavity). The tumor bed is the breast tissue around where the tumor used to be. The remaining breast tissue is the area at next highest risk. Lastly, cancer cells may be trapped in the lymph nodes which drain the breast. These nodes are located in the armpit region (axillary nodes), the low neck near the collarbone (supraclavicular nodes), and behind the breast bone (internal mammary nodes).

Following lumpectomy, radiation may be given to the whole breast (Whole Breast Radiotherapy) or just the lumpectomy cavity (Accelerated Partial Breast Irradiation).

Whole Breast Radiotherapy

Typically, the entire breast is treated after lumpectomy. This is referred to as whole breast irradiation. This portion of treatment usually lasts from 3 to 5 weeks, with treatment delivered once a day, Monday through Friday for a total of 15 to 25 treatments.

Since the area around the lumpectomy cavity is the site at highest risk for recurrence, this area is often given additional radiation treatments. This is referred to as a **boost**. During the boost, the daily dose of radiation is usually kept the same but the radiation is focused on the tumor bed rather than the entire breast. The boost is typically given for an additional 5-8 treatments.

If lymph nodes were found to contain cancer at the time of surgery, then the lymph node areas may also be targeted with radiation. The decision to treat lymph nodes depends on a number of risk factors, including the number and size of lymph nodes involved and the number of nodes removed from the axilla at the time of surgery.

Breast radiotherapy in the United States has traditionally been given once a day over 5-7 weeks. In other countries, shorter courses of 3-4 weeks have been routinely used. These two approaches have been compared head-to-head in research studies. The long-term (>10 year) follow up from these trials has demonstrated that a shorter course of radiation is as effective and safe as the longer course. Short course radiation is usually an option when the lymph nodes are not being treated.

What Types Of Radiation Are Used For Whole Breast Radiation?

When the entire breast or the lymph nodes are being targeted, radiation is always delivered from outside the body. The two main forms of radiation in this setting are **3D conformal radiation therapy** and **intensity modulated radiation therapy.**

3D Conformal Radiotherapy: Prior to beginning treatment, a custom radiation treatment plan must be generated. This starts with a CT scan. This scan is loaded into the treatment planning computer. It is then used to generate a three-dimensional rendering of your body. Next, the physician outlines the areas to target with radiation, as well as normal tissues to avoid (like the heart and lungs). Being able to see where the internal organs are in relation to the target area allows your treatment team to determine the best angles for the radiation beams. Each beam is then shaped to reach the target and avoid normal tissues. This process is referred to as 3D conformal radiotherapy. As the radiation beam exits the machine, it is shaped by small leaves made of tungsten. In this way, the radiation field is shaped to cover the target area while minimizing the radiation dose to other organs.

3D conformal radiation may be performed with either photons or electrons. Both photons and electrons are made by a linear accelerator. Photons are basically high-energy x-rays. Since photons can travel long distances through tissue, the beams for breast radiation are typically arranged in two opposing fields. Radiation from one beam enters from the side of the breast and exits near the breast-bone. Radiation from the other beam enters near the breast-bone and exits out the side of the breast. In this way, radiation to the rest of the body is minimized.

Electron therapy uses charged particles of radiation. Unlike photons, electrons deposit all their energy within several centimeters then stop. This makes them ideally suited for treating surface areas. Electrons are often used to deliver an additional "boost" to the tumor bed following whole breast radiation, but they are not well suited to treatment of the whole breast.

Intensity Modulated Radiation Therapy (IMRT): While 3D conformal radiation therapy controls the shape of the radiation coming from the machine, the amount of radiation is consistent throughout all parts of the beam. In IMRT, the amount of radiation coming from different parts of the beam is adjusted during the treatment. This essentially divides each of the radiation fields into thousands of smaller fields. During the radiation planning process, multiple beams are placed at different angles to converge on the breast tissue or lymph node regions. This includes beams that are entering or exiting through healthy tissues like the heart, lungs, and the other breast. A sophisticated computer program then determines how much radiation to deliver through each part of each field to come up with a plan that meets all of the constraints set by the physician. While IMRT is routine for some types of cancers, it is used less frequently for breast cancer. When multiple different fields are used with IMRT, this technique is very effective at shaping high-dose regions off of the heart. The greatest concern with using IMRT to treat early-stage breast cancer is that larger volumes of healthy organs receive low dose radiation as compared to 3D conformal radiotherapy.

How Would Whole Breast Radiotherapy Affect My Daily Routine?

Radiation is delivered once a day, Monday though Friday. Your treatment is typically given at the same time each day. Each treatment is quick; you are usually in and out of the department in 15 or 20 minutes. After you arrive, the radiation therapists will escort you into the treatment room and onto the treatment table. There, the therapists will help position you appropriately. Most often, this is face up with your arms supported on rests above your head. Once you are properly aligned, radiation treatment can proceed. The machine is usually only delivering radiation for about two minutes. You may hear the machine but you will not see or feel anything during the treatment. Some women report feeling a slight warmth in the breast following treatment. You may also notice some pinkness of the skin of the breast shortly after treatment. Otherwise, you will typically feel the same when you leave the department as you did when you arrived. For some women, side effects from treatment can make it difficult to work. When this happens, it is usually near the end of treatment or several days after the completion of treatment. Most women are able to work and continue with their normal activities throughout the course of treatment.

Accelerated Partial Breast Irradiation (APBI)

In comparison to the multiple weeks of treatment used with whole-breast radiation Accelerated Partial Breast Irradiation (APBI) allows for radiation to be completed over a 5 day period. In APBI, radiation is targeted just to the tissue surrounding the surgical cavity. Since only a small volume of breast tissue is targeted, larger doses of radiation can be safely delivered and the total number of treatments can be reduced. Typically, APBI is given over five days with two treatments given per day, with treatments at least 6 hours apart. Since APBI just targets the lumpectomy cavity, this technique is only used as a stand-alone radiation treatment when there is a low probability of having cancer in other parts of the breast or in the lymph nodes. The use of this treatment option has increased significantly in recent years.

Whole Breast Radiation Versus Partial Breast Radiation?

Whole breast radiation has been the standard treatment following lumpectomy for more than 30 years. While this technique has an established track record, it requires a minimum of three weeks of daily treatment. This schedule can be a significant disruption to a woman's life; whether it is interference with family, the cost of missed work, or the difficulty of traveling to a medical facility every day for several weeks.

Accelerated partial breast irradiation (APBI) was developed to address these issues. APBI allows physicians to precisely deliver treatment to the lumpectomy cavity and surrounding tissue. This reduces treatment time down to five days and reduces radiation dose to healthy tissues.

APBI is a very safe, effective, and convenient form of radiation treatment. Initial research indicates APBI can be as effective as whole breast radiation in select groups of patients. Large, head-to-head trials comparing APBI to whole breast radiation are currently being conducted. These studies will establish whether APBI becomes the standard treatment for most women following lumpectomy. Until these results are available, highly respected national medical societies such as the American Brachytherapy Society (ABS), the American Society of Breast surgeons (ASBS), and the American Society for Radiation Oncology (ASTRO) have set recommendations on which patients are candidates for APBI. If you are interested in learning if you are a candidate for this therapy, please discuss this with your treating physicians.

How Is Accelerated Partial Breast Irradiation (APBI) Performed?

There are two different general approaches to APBI: radiation may be delivered externally (using 3D conformal radiotherapy or IMRT) or it may be delivered from inside the breast (brachytherapy).

Breast brachytherapy: In brachytherapy, flexible hollow plastic tubes called catheters or a balloon are inserted directly into the lumpectomy cavity. The closed ends of the tubes are located in the tumor bed and the open ends come out through the skin of the breast. During treatment, the catheters or the balloon are connected to a machine, which stores a small radioactive pellet, or seed (approximately the size of a grain of rice). With a special computer and robotic control, this small, radioactive seed is guided through the catheters and into the lumpectomy cavity. The radioactive seed is left in place for several minutes until the correct dose of radiation is delivered. When the treatment is complete, the seed is pulled back into the shielded container and the catheter is disconnected from the machine.

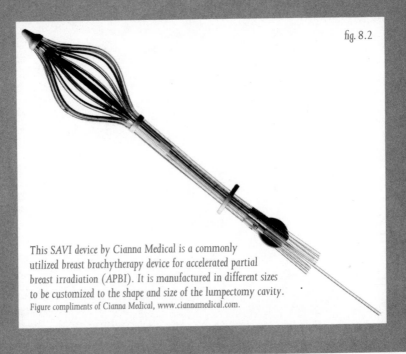

fig. 8.2

This *SAVI* device by Cianna Medical is a commonly utilized breast brachytherapy device for accelerated partial breast irradiation (APBI). It is manufactured in different sizes to be customized to the shape and size of the lumpectomy cavity.
Figure compliments of Cianna Medical, www.ciannamedical.com.

There is no radioactivity left behind after the procedure. This treatment is performed twice a day, at least six hours apart over five total days. After the last treatment, the catheters or balloon are removed very easily.

External beam APBI: This technique uses the same radiation machine utilized for whole breast radiotherapy. In external beam APBI, multiple radiation beams are used to target the lumpectomy cavity. Treatment may be performed using 3D conformal or IMRT techniques. This treatment is also typically given twice daily over five days.

fig. 8.3

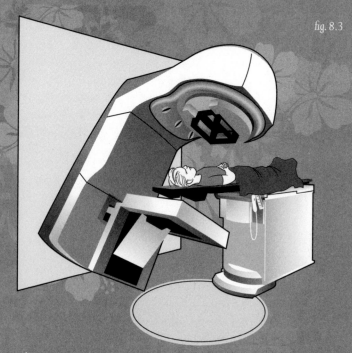

Linear accelerators are machines that can precisely focus high energy x-ray beams. These machines have been traditionally used to treat the whole breast, and more recently have been used for external beam accelerated partial breast irradiation.

Who Is A Candidate For APBI?

This is a treatment option that needs to be discussed in depth with your cancer treatment team. Most established guidelines by national oncology groups include patients who:

1. Are older than age 45-50

2. Have small tumor sizes measuring less than 2-3 cm diameter

3. Have a lumpectomy with negative surgical margins and no lymph nodes involved

4. Do not have the pathology features of "extensive intraductal component" or "lymphovascular space invasion" (examined by a pathologist)

5. Have pathologic "ductal carcinoma" type of cancer [some national guidelines also include Ductal Carcinoma in Situ (DCIS)]*

How Would "Accelerated Partial Breast Irradiation" Affect My Daily Routine?

For APBI, radiation is given twice daily for five days with treatments spaced at least six hours apart. The time required for each treatment varies depending on the radiation technique but generally each treatment can be completed in less than 30 minutes. For women receiving brachytherapy, the medical device remains in the breast during the entire course of treatment (1 week), so patients must refrain from showering during this time. The device is carefully secured with gauze to minimize movement between treatments. Many women report minimal disruption to their daily lives. While some women choose to take time off from work and other activities, others report that they were able to carry on their normal schedules during the course of treatment.

Following brachytherapy treatment, the most common side effects are temporary redness, bruising and discomfort. These do not occur in all patients. Most women find it possible to resume their normal daily activities immediately following treatment.

*Guideline information obtained from the American Brachytherapy Society (ABS) and the American Society of Breast Surgeons (ASBS).[1]

When Is Radiation Given Following Mastectomy?

Because mastectomy removes all of the breast tissue, this type of surgery significantly decreases the chance of the cancer returning on that side. Still, even after mastectomy, the cancer may return on the chest wall (where the breast used to sit) or in the lymph nodes. Several factors are used to determine how likely the cancer is to return after mastectomy. The main factors are whether or not the cancer has spread to the lymph nodes, how many lymph nodes are involved, the original size of the tumor, how responsive the tumor is to chemotherapy, and how the tumor looks under the microscope. Sometimes, the risk of the cancer returning after mastectomy and chemotherapy is very low (<5%). In these cases, radiation may not be recommended due to the small benefit and potential side effects of treatment.

What Types Of Radiation Are Used Following Mastectomy?

The radiation techniques used most frequently after mastectomy are 3D conformal radiotherapy and IMRT. These techniques are also used following lumpectomy and are described in detail on page 65.

Following a mastectomy, the area at highest risk for recurrence is the skin overlying the chest wall, followed by the lymph nodes. Sometimes, a sheet of special material called a bolus is placed on the skin during radiation. This material increases the radiation dose at the skin surface to ensure that any cancer cells remaining in the skin are killed. The radiation to the chest wall typically lasts for 5 weeks, with treatment delivered once per day, Monday through Friday, for a total of 25 to 30 treatments. Additional radiation may be directed to areas at increased risk for recurrence. This portion of the treatment, called the "boost", typically lasts for an additional 5 to 8 treatments. Just as with radiation following lumpectomy, radiation may also be directed at the axilla, supraclavicular, or substernal regions in order to treat the lymph nodes where breast cancer is most likely to spread.

Special Considerations Following Mastectomy

After mastectomy, there are various cosmetic options. Some patients choose to use a breast prosthesis which fits in a bra. Others choose to have additional surgery to reconstruct the breast. Breast reconstruction falls into two general categories: implant based or autologous tissue based. An implant reconstruction uses a saline or silicone device placed underneath the skin. In autologous reconstruction, the plastic surgeon uses your own tissue to reconstruct the breast. This tissue may be taken from the abdomen or back. Radiation can be performed either before or after reconstruction. However, implant based reconstruction may be more difficult to perform after radiation therapy.

It is important to discuss reconstruction options early with your surgeon. If prior to surgery, it is known that radiation will be necessary, a temporary tissue expander may be placed under the skin at the time of mastectomy. A tissue expander essentially acts as a spacer to stretch the skin and prevent scar tissue from forming between the skin and the chest wall. This may increase reconstruction options. After surgery, the expander is filled with saline over a series of visits. Once the expander is fully expanded, radiation is performed. Several months after radiation is complete, the expander is removed and a final surgery is performed.

When Is Radiation Used For Metastatic Cancer?

Once cancer has spread (metastasized) beyond lymph nodes to other organs, it is not generally considered curable. Despite this, patients with metastatic breast cancer can live many years with little or no symptoms. In this setting, radiation is most often used after cancer has spread to a bone or to the brain. Palliative radiation is very effective at relieving pain and preventing fractures. On average, radiation for bone pain is more than 80% effective. Radiation for tumors that have spread to the brain can extend life and also slow or prevent the development of neurologic symptoms.

What Types Of Radiation Are Used For Whole Breast Radiation And After Mastectomy?

The techniques used for whole breast radiation and after mastectomy are similar. When the entire breast or the lymph nodes are being targeted, radiation is always delivered from outside the body. The two main forms of radiation in this setting are 3D conformal radiation therapy and intensity modulated radiation therapy.

3D Conformal Radiotherapy

The type of radiation treatment used most frequently for breast cancer is 3D conformal therapy. After simulation, the CT scan taken at the simulation is loaded into the treatment planning computer. It is then used to generate a three-dimensional rendering of your body. Next, the physician outlines the areas to target with radiation, as well as normal tissues to avoid (like the heart and lungs). Being able to see where the internal organs are in relation to the target area allows your treatment team to determine the best angles for the radiation beams. Each beam is then shaped to reach the target and avoid normal tissues. This process is referred to as 3D conformal radiotherapy. As the radiation beam exits the machine, it is shaped by small leaves made of tungsten metal. In this way, the radiation field is shaped to cover the target area while minimizing the radiation dose to other organs.

3D conformal radiation may be performed with either photons or electrons. Both photons and electrons are made by a linear accelerator. Photons are basically high-energy x-rays. Since photons can travel long distances through tissue, the beams for breast radiation are typically arranged in two opposing fields. Radiation from one beam enters from the side of the breast and exits near the breast-bone. Radiation from the other beam enters near the breast bone and exits out the side of the breast. In this way, radiation to the rest of the body (deeper tissue) is minimized.

Electron therapy uses charged particles of radiation. Unlike photons, electrons deposit all their energy within the first few centimeters then stop. This makes them ideally suited for treating surface areas. Electrons are often used to deliver an additional "boost" to the tumor bed following whole breast radiation, but they are not well suited to treatment of the whole breast.

Intensity Modulated Radiation Therapy (IMRT)

Intensity modulated radiation therapy (IMRT) is similar to 3D conformal radiation therapy. With IMRT in addition to shaping the radiation beam, the intensity of the radiation within each beam is varied. IMRT uses the metal leaves in the machine to basically divide each beam into thousands of smaller beamlets. In this way, the intensity of radiation coming through each part of the beam can be varied. When IMRT is used with multiple beam angles, the physician, with the help of specialized computers, determines how much radiation dose to deliver through each beamlet. This allows the high dose radiation to be focused tightly on the target and spare nearby organs. While IMRT is routine for some types of cancers, it is not frequently used for breast cancer. The greatest concern with using IMRT to treat breast cancer is that larger volumes of healthy organs receive low dose radiation as compared to 3D conformal radiotherapy. (see pg. 66)

What Types Of Radiation Are Used For Partial Breast Irradiation?

When only a small portion of the breast is being targeted for treatment, radiation may delivered externally (using 3D conformal radiotherapy or IMRT) or it may be delivered from inside the breast. Internal radiation may be delivered in several different ways. Treatment delivered by placing a radioactive device or radioactive material inside the body is called brachytherapy.

IntraOperative Radiation Therapy (IORT)

IntraOperative Radiation Therapy (IORT) is a technique in which radiation is delivered directly to the breast tissue around where the tumor used to be, called the tumor bed, at the time of surgery. IORT may minimize the amount of normal tissues receiving radiation and may allow for all of the treatment to be completed at the time of surgery. IORT is currently under investigation as a substitute for conventional radiation in patients at low risk for having additional sites of microscopic cancer.

What Types Of Radiation Are Used For Metastatic Cancer?

The technique used to treat metastatic cancer depends on the location of the tumor and whether radiation has previously been used to treat a nearby area. The most frequently used technique is 3D conformal radiation. If radiation therapy has already been used in the past, it is important to limit the dose to organs that previously received radiation. Although tissues usually recover completely from a course of radiation, there are maximum limits for how much dose each organ can receive over a lifetime. IMRT is especially useful for avoiding areas of prior radiation. In some situations, radiation for metastatic tumors can also be performed with Stereotactic Radiotherapy.

Stereotactic Radiotherapy (SRT)

Stereotactic radiotherapy is a precise form of treatment in which very high doses of radiation are given to a small area. In stereotactic radiotherapy, the tumor is targeted from multiple beam angles. All of the radiation beams meet at the tumor. In this way, the dose of radiation coming in through the normal tissues can be kept to safe levels while delivering a very high dose within the tumor itself. Stereotactic radiotherapy is often given as a single treatment for a tumor that has spread to the brain. In this case, it is referred to as Stereotactic RadioSurgery (SRS). GammaKnife is a dedicated machine used to treat many types of brain tumors with SRS.

When body sites other than the brain are treated, it is called stereotactic body radiotherapy (SBRT). While there are numerous different types of machines capable of performing stereotactic radiotherapy (SRT), Specialized Linear Accelerators and Cyberknife are designed specifically for SBRT. SBRT is dependent more upon the physician's experience than on the type of machine used.

What Tests Are Necessary Before Deciding On
A Final Treatment Strategy?

Prior to starting treatment, your doctor may order additional tests. The goal of these tests is to determine if the cancer has spread to other parts of the body. Depending on your stage of cancer, certain blood tests may be useful. These tests most often measure liver activity or bone turnover which may be increased if the cancer has spread. While there is no specific blood test for detecting breast cancer in everyone, certain tumors do make substances that are detectable in the blood. These "tumor markers" are helpful for tracking whether treatment is effective. The most common tumor marker in breast cancer is CA 27–29.

Depending on the stage of the cancer, additional imaging studies may also be helpful. If there is a high risk that your cancer might spread, your doctor may recommend a bone scan, PET/CT, or an MRI scan. Each test has certain strengths and drawbacks.

A bone scan is used for determining whether cancer has spread to the bones. When breast cancer spreads to bone, it typically causes the bone to try to grow or repair itself. This is called remodeling. For the bone scan, a small amount of radioactive substance is injected into the vein. This substance is taken up by bone that is remodeling itself and shows up as a bright spot on the bone scan. However, arthritis and old injuries can also cause bone remodeling which can show up on a bone scan.

A PET scan (Positron Emission Tomography) is also a nuclear study. For this test, a small amount of radioactive sugar is injected into the vein. This sugar is taken up by tissues that are metabolically active. Cancer cells, which tend to be rapidly dividing compared to surrounding tissues, appear bright on the PET scan. However, other tissues that are metabolically active (such as the brain) and areas of inflammation (from surgery or infection) can also appear bright on a PET scan. A PET scan combined with a CT scan (PET/CT) at the same time helps precisely locate areas of disease within the body.

It is important to recognize that no test is 100% effective at detecting cancer. Imaging studies cannot detect individual cancer cells. Additionally, there is always a chance that something will be detected on a scan that looks like cancer, but is not cancer. In other words, tests like a bone scan or PET/CT can show a false positive result. For these reasons, these tests should only be performed when there is a high risk that the cancer has spread.

What Steps Are Necessary Before Radiation Treatment Can Begin?

Before radiation can begin, a custom treatment plan needs to be made for you. The preparation of your treatment plan begins with what is called a **simulation**. During the simulation, measurements are made and a special CT scan is taken. This CT scan provides a map of your body which is then used to generate a customized radiation plan. For this procedure, you will lie down on a special table and be placed in the same position that will be used for the actual treatment. The goal is to find a position that you can comfortably maintain during your daily treatments and that allows the radiation beam to avoid as much healthy tissue as possible. This is typically lying on your back with your arms above your head. In some cases, radiation may be performed in the face down, or prone, position, allowing the breast to hang down. A custom body mold may be made to help hold you in the right position during daily treatment.

Once you are in the proper position, a CT scan is taken. In the final step, several small tattoos are placed on your skin. These tattoos provide reference points for the radiation therapists during treatment. Every day when you come in for treatment, you will be placed in the same position that you were in for the simulation and the tattoos will be aligned to lasers in the room. This ensures that the radiation goes exactly where it's supposed to. After the simulation, the doctor works with the medical dosimetrist and specialized computer soft-

Nurse's Note:

Ask about the short and long-term effects of treatment. Some treatments have effects that can be noticed months or years later.

ware to develop a treatment plan. Once a final plan has been approved, it is reviewed by a medical physicist who verifies that everything is correct before starting treatment.

What Are The Side Effects Of Radiation Therapy?

Breast radiation therapy can cause short-term and long-term side effects. While short-term side effects such as fatigue and skin irritation are common, more serious side effects are rare. Some side effects, such as shrinkage of the treated breast, may be long-term.

Short Term Side Effects

The most common short-term side effects during breast radiation therapy are fatigue and skin irritation. Most side effects are cumulative. You usually won't notice much of an effect from a single treatment, but after a week of treatment or more has passed, you may begin to feel these effects.

Most patients will experience some degree of fatigue or tiredness from the radiation treatment. Unlike other side effects, which generally get worse as treatment progresses, fatigue may get better or worse throughout the course of treatment. For most patients, the fatigue from radiation is bothersome but not debilitating. For example, most patients are able to drive themselves to and from treatments. Staying active may minimize the effects of fatigue. Sometimes fatigue may affect your sleep cycle. If you find yourself taking naps through the day and having difficulty sleeping at night, it may be helpful to limit naps to 30 minutes. Also, try to do some physical activity outdoors during the day if possible. Do not get in bed until you are ready to sleep. Acupuncture has been shown to help minimize fatigue associated with breast cancer treatment. Fatigue usually goes away within a month after treatment but for some patients, it may take several months for their energy to completely recover.

Skin irritation occurs in nearly all patients receiving breast radiotherapy. This can vary from slight pinkness of the skin to

Nurse's Note:
Your nurse will give you creams and lotions and direction on their use. This will be important to minimize skin reactions from radiation.

extensive moist peeling resembling a burn. Most patients will begin to notice some pinkness of the skin of the breast after the second or third week of treatment. By the final week of treatment, most patients will experience pinkness throughout the breast, similar to a sunburn. About 25% of women will have peeling of the skin of the breast or chest wall by the end of treatment. This is usually limited to the fold of skin beneath the breast and the armpit area.

Skin care is important during treatment. You should avoid any additional irritation to the skin receiving radiation. Wear a soft padded bra or try not wearing a bra if possible. Wash the skin daily using a mild soap (like Dove). After bathing, pat the area dry with a soft towel. Do not rub. After drying off, apply a mild lotion to the skin. This can be used once or twice daily. Avoid band-aids, strong tapes or adhesives. Try to minimize sun exposure to the area receiving radiation. Be aware that the radiation field for the breast often comes up the collarbone. When lymph nodes are treated, the radiation field comes up the neck.

Although there have been many studies of different creams and lotions, most studies have shown they have little benefit over a simple moisturizer. When choosing a moisturizer, the most important thing is that you are not allergic to it. If you are trying a lotion you've never used before, try it on another area before applying it to the skin receiving radiation. Look for a lotion that is hypo-allergenic, does not have sunscreen and does not have strong fragrance or perfumes. Aloe Vera gel can also be used but sometimes it can get sticky after repeated applications. Petroleum based ointments (Aquaphor) last longer on the skin but some patients find it too greasy. Lotion containing marigold extract (Calendula) may minimize skin irritation during radiation treatment. There are many suitable products. Steroid cream (hydrocortisone) is helpful for itching. If you develop moist skin peeling, petrolatum ointment or silver sulfadiazine may be used. Typically, you will see your radiation oncologist weekly and you can review your side effects and potential treatments during those visits.

During the radiation, you may also have swelling of the breast or discomfort. This is typically controlled with an over the counter anti-inflammatory such as ibuprofen.

After the last radiation treatment, the skin irritation usually plateaus for about 7-10 days before subsiding. Typically, by one month after treatment the skin is healed. At this point, there is usually tanning of the skin that previously was red. This tanning can last several months.

Long-Term Side Effects

The most common long-term side effect of radiation is shrinkage of the treated breast. This can take up to 1-2 years to fully develop. Radiation to the lymph nodes increases the risk of long term swelling of the arm or lymphedema. It is important to be evaluated early for lymphedema. A lymphedema therapist can instruct you on special massages and exercises. Radiation to the lymph nodes can also cause stiffness of the shoulder joint. If you received radiation to the lymph nodes, regular stretching exercises can help maintain your range of motion. Some women have chest wall tenderness. There is a very small risk of developing pneumonitis (inflammation of the lung) on the side treated within 6 months after radiation. The ribs under the treated breast are at a slightly increased risk of fractures. Long-term heart side effects are greatly reduced by the ability to shield the heart better than in the past.

All forms of radiation exposure can increase your lifetime risk of developing a cancer. When radiation therapy is given to the breast or chest wall after cancer surgery, there is a very small risk that the treatment will cause a cancer. At the same time, this treatment is highly effective at preventing the original cancer from returning. The end result is that radiation therapy for breast cancer significantly reduces the overall chance of having cancer in the future.

What Is The Follow-Up After Radiation Treatment?

After radiation, you will continue to have regular follow-up appointments with members of the breast cancer team. During these appointments, your doctor will evaluate for side effects of treatment and look for any evidence that the cancer has returned. Typically, the same tests that were used to detect the cancer originally are used to monitor for recurrence. Please be sure to follow your physician's instructions regarding follow-up appointments or additional treatments specific to your circumstances.

1. Vicini F, Arthur D, Wazer D, et al. Limitations of the American Society of Therapeutic Radiology and Oncology Consensus Panel guidelines on the use of accelerated partial breast irradiation. Int J Radiat Oncol Biol Phys. 2011;79(4):977-84. Epub 2010 May 25.

Beitsch P, Vicini F, Keisch M, Haffty B, Shaitelman S, Lyden M. Five-year outcome of patients classified in the "unsuitable" category using the American Society of Therapeutic Radiology and Oncology (ASTRO) Consensus Panel Guidelines for the Applications of Accelerated Partial Breast Irradiation: an analysis of patients treated on the American Society of Breast Surgeons MammoSite® Registry Trial. Ann Surg Oncol. 2010;17(Suppl3):S219-25.

McHaffie DR, Patel RR, Adkison JB, et al. Outcomes after accelerated partial breast irradiation in patients with ASTRO consensus statement cautionary features. Int J Radiat Oncol Biol Phys. 2011;81(1):46-51.

Shaitelman SF, Vicini FA, Beitsch PPD, et al. Time to revise the consensus statement guidelines for the use of accelerated partial breast irradiation off protocol. Int J Radiat Oncol Biol Phys. 2011;81(Suppl):S204

Jeruss JS, Kuerer HM, Beitsch PD, Vicini FA, Keisch M. Update on DCIS outcomes from the American Society of Breast Surgeons accelerated partial breast irradiation registry trial. Ann Surg Oncol. 2011;18(1):65-71. Epub 2010 Jun 25.

Part Nine

Focusing On Nutrition

"Breast cancer." Two words that can change your world. "You have breast cancer." Four words that can cause your life to flash before your eyes. It's unsettling to say the least. Many patients come in feeling desperate and at a loss, but it is those same patients that grab cancer by the tail and say, "Hey, I'm not going to let cancer bully me. It's time to fight and I am going to do what I can to beat you or at the very least, control you so I can live my life!" Following some nutritional and

fig. 9.1

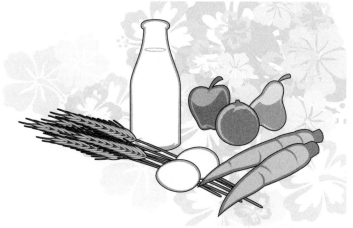

Focusing on nutrition can be the best thing that you can do for yourself during cancer therapy.

lifestyle recommendations can help in fighting breast cancer. Some things that can help make you feel a little more in control of what may feel like an out of control situation are laid out on the following pages. What you choose to eat can have a strong impact on fighting this cancer. Your immune system is what fights off illnesses and disease. By making the best choices nutritionally, you can maximize your immune system's fighting potential, making you the best cancer fighter you can be. It's all about boosting your immune system, fighting inflammation and decreasing challenges to your immune system so it can focus on the current battle at hand.

Knowledge is power. It's time to empower you with knowledge in this fight against cancer. Use it to arm yourself with knowledge. Let's get to it!

American Institute Of Cancer Research (AICR) Findings-Breast Cancer:

Visit **AICR.org** or **foodandcancerreport.org** to download, for free, the findings from the 2007, 2nd Expert Report. The information provided by the AICR expert report was broken down into two sections for breast cancer. The evidence and judgments were divided into "pre-menopause" and "post-menopause".

There is convincing evidence that lactation decreases risk of breast cancer, and intake of alcoholic drinks increases risk regardless if one is either pre or post-menopause. There is probable evidence that body fatness decreases risk during pre-menopausal period, while body fatness, post-menopause, increases risk of breast cancer. The reason being the body fat distribution that occurs with menopause is mainly in the abdominal area. There is apparently more visceral fat (inside the abdominal cavity) which harbors those toxins and harmful substances. It is also known that a waistline of >35 inches for females is a risk factor for cancers, heart disease and other diseases. Physical activity/exercise decrease risk of breast cancer both pre and post-menopause.

What are you supposed to do with this information? Well, basically, this means to eat more foods that are anti-inflammatory, immune boosting, lower in fat, and mostly plant based, and drink less or no alcohol. Physical activity is a must as well. Specific foods are found to be more anti-inflammatory than others, which is why a variety of nutritional intake is recommended. A couple of powerful nutrients are selenium and quercitin, which are referred to as flavonoids, or more specifically flavonols. Selenium is found more in certain nuts and seeds and fish, while flavonols are found in vegetables and darker colored fruits. Both selenium and quercitin are naturally occurring antioxidants and are anti-inflammatory. Please see below for lists of foods containing these flavonoids. Intake of these foods are encouraged, but please talk to your doctor, naturopathic doctor, or dietitian about taking quercitin supplementation.

As for the physical activity recommendations, get moving more! Be more active and get that blood pumping! Physical activity helps directly and indirectly to decrease cancer risk. Also, it can improve mental state or mood, release negative energy and help fight inflammation. The federal guidelines for exercise are great and relatively easy to attain. It is recommended we get physically active at least 150 minutes a week or do 75 minutes a week of vigorous exercise each week. In addition to that, you should do weight training (just about 15 minutes) twice a week. See!? You can do this! It may not be so easy if you are undergoing treatment and are fatigued, however, try to be as active as possible to help maintain muscle mass. One important rule to follow during your treatment is to listen to your body. Monitor your fatigue level and just do what you can. Resistance bands are great for helping you to keep muscle tone and can be done while sitting in the comforts of your own home. You must be careful if you have recently undergone surgery for breast or tumor removal, and please note if you have any signs of lymphedema you should talk to a physical therapist specialized in this area about the amount of movement that is allowed, to safely avoid making lymphedema any worse.

Nurse's Note:

Always consult your doctor before starting a new exercise program.

Alcohol intake should be limited, or none at all. WHAT!?!? "What about that glass of wine every night I have while making dinner?!" you ask. Well, that should be OK. For females, one, 6 ounce glass of wine is considered "in moderation". Some of you right now are screaming, "More like a drop!" But when looking at the information there is convincing evidence to support such recommendations. Sincerely think about decreasing intake of wine and other alcoholic beverages.

Another recommendation is to decrease body fatness by decreasing the amount of inflammatory fats consumed and increasing that physical activity level. Read on and more detailed information on kinds of fats to consume and more powerful information on immune boosting nutrition is ahead.

Selenium Containing Foods:

- Brazil nuts
- Sunflower seeds
- Tuna (canned light tuna in oil)
- Cod (cooked)

Quercitin Containing Foods:

- Apples
- Red or black grapes
- Blueberries
- Blackberries
- Cherries
- Onions (raw yields 30% more quercitin than cooked)
- Scallions
- Kale
- Broccoli
- Green tea and red wine from dark grapes (as stated by Linus Pauling Institute)

Go to **livestrong.com** for more information on quercitin if you like.

IMMUNE BOOSTING NUTRITION

Make every bite count. Well, almost every bite. Follow the 80/20 rule. Eighty percent of the time you should make every bite count. Make the best choice for what you decide to fuel your body with. So often we are on the go, or in a hurry, and making unconscious decisions regarding our nutritional intake. Think about it. Is what you are eating doing anything for your body and your fight against cancer? If not, maybe you should think about making some changes in your food selections. That's not to say you can't enjoy those foods that, let's be honest, aren't good for you but they sure taste good and make you feel happy. You can. These are the foods that you have only around 20% of the time. Enjoying birthday celebrations, dessert out with girlfriends, or any number of social occasions, will most likely involve chips, dips and drink choices that you seldom consume. It's OK to enjoy these moments. Make a conscious effort to eat the best you can most of the time, so you can enjoy these special moments and the "not so good" nutrition choices that accompany these occasions without the guilt. It's all part of a healthy eating experience. It's all part of life, as is this current fight you've got on your hands.

Mainly, regarding your diet, the focus should lie on getting back to the basics. Having less processed foods is where it's at! When buying boxed/convenience foods, select those with less ingredients. Take ice cream for example. It can be a source of protein and calcium, but has high content of fat, therefore, only consume it occasionally. What you should look at, though, is how many ingredients went into making it. Buy the ice cream containing only five ingredients or so. Breyers All Natural is a good example of this. This is not saying eat ice cream all the time, but it is okay sometimes, especially if there are no chemicals/preservatives added to it. This was just an example. In general, focus on eating whole grains, dark and brightly colored fruits and vegetables, plant proteins, lean animal protein sources, fish (especially those high in Omega-3 fatty acids), and other good fats which are listed below. The idea is to balance out carbs and protein at each meal, mini meal or snack. Also by incorporating the good fats into your diet, this will help in sparing the protein you take in for healing and repair.

Whole Grains

When choosing whole grain foods, select those that have been the least processed or are closer to their natural state. Some examples of whole grains include: brown rice, wild rice, whole wheat pasta, quinoa, quinoa pasta, high fiber cereals (hot or cold) containing 5 grams or more fiber per serving, and breads made from whole grain flour, having 3 grams of fiber or more per slice. Whole grain flour being the first ingredient listed. Whole grains have complex carbohydrates in them which are needed by our bodies for energy. They also have protein in them. Quinoa, for example, has 6-10 grams of protein per ½ cup. Give it a try if you haven't already.

Produce

It is recommended that 5 or more servings of fruit and vegetables be consumed each day. This is challenging for a lot of people. A recommendation that is easy to adhere to is to add a fruit or vegetable to every meal, mini meal or snack eaten during the day. Try to eat small meals, every 3 hours or so. At each of these add a serving of produce. Aim for 5 servings a day of dark or brightly colored produce.

Some Of The Best Choices Include:

• **Broccoli, cauliflower, brussels sprouts, kale and bok choy.** These are called cruciferous vegetables and they contain isothiocyanates, specifically Indole-3-Carbinol. This is a cancer fighting compound and should be consumed on a daily basis!

• **Berries** of all varieties.

• **Carrots** and orange colored produce for the carotenoids. (Carotenoid-containing foods are especially good for fighting breast cancer!)

- **Red grapes** for the resveratrol.

- **Green leafies**.

- **Tomatoes**.

This is a short list of some of the most powerful cancer fighting produce available at grocery stores. It is highly recommended you have your own garden if you can, and grow produce organically. Another thing that should always be mentioned when discussing produce is to wash it in a vinegar and water solution. Wash produce using a solution of 1 Tablespoon vinegar (any kind) in 4 cups of water. This will help to pull off 95-99% of the cancer-causing pesticides used in the farming of the produce. For the thin skinned fruits and hard to wash vegetables, it is better to go organic because it is difficult to completely clean these off. This decreases challenges to your immune system, one less thing to worry about.

Plant Proteins

Foods of plant origin are high in fiber, vitamins, minerals, antioxidants, beneficial plant compounds, and prebiotic fibers to help support healthy intestinal bacteria balance. Plant based foods are the basis for an anti-inflammatory diet. Beans, legumes, lentils, nuts, seeds, soy foods—these are all sources of protein coming from a plant source. GO FOR IT! Add these to your salads, soups, chilies, or make a bean burger, etc.

Animal Proteins

Protein from animal sources is allowed also, but be sure to buy leaner cuts of meat, chicken and other poultry with no skin, and go organic when it comes to purchasing red meat and dairy products containing fat. Buy grass fed cattle because it is higher in Omega-3 fatty acids which are anti-inflammatory. Animal foods, in general, contain higher amount of Omega-6 fatty acids which are pro-inflammatory so the goal is to decrease intake of animal based foods, and increase

*Freezing your favor-
ite foods may help
you plan your meals
in advance.*

intake of plant based foods and fish, especially those high in Omega-3 fats (sources listed below). Why avoid processed/cured meats? They contain nitrates/nitrite which are known to cause cancer. This cancer causing agent is used in hams, deli meats, hot dogs, bacon and sausages. Select nitrate-free products such as Hormel Natural Selections deli meat, bacon, etc and limit intake. It can be found in the deli meat section of the grocery store.

List Of Protein Foods:

Beans, legumes, lentils – Typical serving size is ¼ cup which equals 7 grams protein. Increase bean intake – try hummus spread, made from garbanzo beans (aka chickpeas).

Nuts, seeds – ¼ cup = 7 grams protein. If nuts and seeds are not tolerated, grind nuts into a spread at your local grocery store. The nut grinders are usually found in the "Health Food" section of the grocery stores by the "All Natural" items.

Soy foods are considered safe for all breast cancer patients to a certain degree. One to three servings of soy foods are allowed for breast cancer patients who are estrogen receptor positive (ER+). What is not recommended are the concentrated forms of soy, such as soy protein powders and soy protein isolates found in many energy bars and meal replacement drinks. Some examples of serving sizes of soy foods include: 1 cup soy milk, 4 ounces tofu, 1/3 cup soy nuts, 6 ounces soy yogurt, ½ cup textured vegetable protein and 1 cup edamame (in pod). It would be okay to have 1-3 servings/day of these soy foods.

Milks and spreads/nut butter made from plant foods – Almond milk, soy milk, soy yogurt, or may grind any nut to make a nut butter at your local grocery store. (Please note as stated previously, intake of soy foods considered safe at 1-3 servings/day if breast cancer is hormone receptor positive (ER+/PR+). A serving size of a nut butter is typically 2 tablespoons.

Fish – Especially wild caught salmon, tuna, halibut, mackerel and rainbow trout, for their Omega-3 fatty acid content. Omega-3s, as stated previously, are a natural anti-inflammatory and should be consumed 2-3 times per week. Other fish do not contain high levels of Omega-3s, however, are lean protein sources, 4 ounces being a serving of fish it provides 28 grams of protein. High mercury levels have been found in marine sources, so it is suggested to eat fish only 2-3 times per week. Omega-3 supplementation is recommended for this reason.

Eggs are a high quality protein. Each egg has about 5-7 grams of protein. Suggest having 5 eggs a week and unlimited egg whites.

Chicken and turkey – No skin, are lean protein sources. Each ounce has 7 grams protein.

LEAN cuts of red meat – Sirloin, ground sirloin for burgers vs. ground chuck, and flank steak for fajitas, for example, would be okay for consumption. Also, look for grass-fed cattle as this meat will have more Omega-3s vs the inflammatory Omega-6s. The AICR generally recommends limiting intake of red meat, to about 3 servings per week.

Greek yogurt has about 12-14 grams protein in it and four to five different strains of live cultures (probiotics) which will help to normalize gut flora and promote bacteria balance in the intestines.

Low or no-fat dairy – Skim milk, 1% milk, low fat, skim mozzarella, etc. When buying a fat-containing animal product it is recommended to go organic. Look for the following statement or something similar on the label, "No hormones or antibiotics were given to this animal or used in the making of this product." Keep in mind when buying fat-containing animal foods: hormones, and toxins given to the animal are stored in the fat of the animal (Much like humans). The fattier the animal food, the more likely you are to consume the bad things stored in the fat of the animal. Safer to go organic when it comes to fat-containing animal products. It is wise to spend your money on organic meats and dairy products.

Good Fats

Lowering dietary intake of Omega-6 fats (mostly animal foods) while raising intake of Omega-3 fats will help to shift the body into "anti-inflammatory" mode. What are good sources of Omega-3s? High Omega-3 foods include wild caught salmon, tuna, halibut, mackerel and rainbow trout. Also, foods of plant origin will have less Omega-6 fats and some Omega-3s like walnuts and flaxseed oil. Extra virgin olive oil, canola oil and coconut oil are examples of good fats as are avocados, nuts and seeds. Daily intake of a ¼ - ½ of an avocado is recommended.

Hydration

Keeping the body hydrated is so very important every day, not just during treatment for cancer. You, in general, need 13-18 ml of non-caloric, caffeine free fluids per pound of weight each day to maintain a good hydration status. Example: 150 lbs x 13 ml/lb = 1950 ml/day which is equivalent to 8 ¼ cups per day of fluid. Monitor urine frequency, color and odor. If it looks concentrated or darker in color and has an odor, you very well may be dehydrated. On the day of chemotherapy you will receive one liter of fluid with treatment to assure you are adequately hydrated and that the chemo is flushed through your kidneys appropriately. On the other days, it is all up to you to maintain your fluid intake. If you find yourself having trouble getting enough fluid in, be sure to inform your oncologist, nurse and/or dietitian to possibly get set up for IV fluids a few days a week. Hydration is that important! It is just as important as food intake. The more vocal you are with your symptoms, the better they can be managed, so inform your healthcare team early and often. And work on staying hydrated as best as you can! Another thing you need to work hard on is consistent food intake all day long to fuel your body for cancer fighting!

BALANCE, TIMING, And PLANNING All To Regulate Blood Sugar And Keep The Body Fueled!

Fueling your body consistently all day long, every day, will help to maintain an even keel throughout the day and avoid peaks and valleys associated with varying sugar intake. By staying on an even keel all day you will provide needed support to your immune system so that it can work at its best potential. Blood sugar stabilization is key. Statements like,

"I don't eat breakfast." Or, "My whole life I've never eaten breakfast", are often heard and now is the time for that to change. Try to consume calories, whether it's eating or drinking, within an hour of waking. You need to wake the body up and let it know that nutrition is on the way. If you're not doing this, it is very likely that your metabolism will slow down. Another very important thing to remember is that caffeine is an appetite suppressant. Countless people have said, "I just drink black coffee all morning and I'm not hungry for anything until about 4:00 in the afternoon." The reason one can go so long without having an appetite is due, in part, to the caffeine intake as it is an appetite suppressant—not signaling the hunger cue. In actuality, you are slowing down the metabolism. What you need now is a well-oiled machine and to stay revved up to support weight maintenance as well as your immune system. We are addressing weight management and immune-boosting nutrition. To continue boosting the immune system and support your cancer fighting body, eating every 3 hours is suggested, trying never to go longer than 4 hours between intake. This will help to support blood sugar stability all day long and keep you and your immune system energized.

Imagine this: your body is a wood stove. You want to keep the fire burning all day long so you need logs (protein foods) and kindling (carbohydrates) every few hours. Why do this? The answer is simple. If your body doesn't have consistent source of fuel, it will think, "Uh-oh, I don't have anything coming in", and begin to work its magic in fueling your body, slowing things down if you will and eventually pulling from energy stores in your body. You have stored energy in your muscles and when not properly nourished you may begin to breakdown muscle. A good way to gauge muscle loss is to look at your arms. Look for atrophy (shrinking muscle mass). Notice if there is any muscle or fat loss. Of course, monitor your weight. It is okay to lose a little bit of weight but want to avoid significant weight loss. Your oncologist and care team will be following you during and after your treatment to monitor your overall health status. Significant weight loss is indicative of the inability to meet caloric needs. The registered dietitian on the team will be alerted if you should experience significant weight loss, change in nutritional status, and/or begin to be more symptomatic. A nutrition consult would be beneficial to address and possibly prevent or minimize symptoms you may encounter and provide you with ways to manage them. Managing side effects early can help to minimize the symptoms, thus minimizing the impact they may have on your overall nutritional status. It is very important to let your physician, nurse, dietitian, or any member of the healthcare team know of any or all symptoms you may be experiencing.

SYMPTOMS

Symptoms associated with treatment for breast cancer include: constipation (from pain meds, mostly), diarrhea, decreased or no appetite, sore throat, painful swallowing, difficulty swallowing, taste changes, nausea, vomiting, and anemia. Hair loss may occur and for some breast cancer patients, this is one of the most dreaded of symptoms simply because there is a feeling of vulnerability associated with hair loss. It is commonly stated that one doesn't wish to appear sick and when they lose their hair, it may become apparent to others that something is going on. There are many resources and people to contact regarding use of wigs, accessories and other boutique items. Be sure to talk with the social worker/ case manager or patient navigator to get familiar with all that is available to you in your community.

Esophagitis may occur if radiation is part of the treatment and the location of the tumor is near the esophagus. Oftentimes, radiation therapy will be used to shrink the tumor and if the tumor is located near the esophagus, it may cause painful swelling of the esophageal area. Esophagitis is inflammation of the esophagus and can make it painful or difficult in getting foods all the way down. During radiation the body will naturally send lubrication to the site of radiation, as well as send inflammation to this site in attempts to heal. Sure the body is trying to heal this area, but it can make it difficult to swallow when there is inflammation in and around the esophagus. To manage the lubrication, which may be in the form of a sticky, thick, mucus-like phlegm, it is best to stay hydrated. Drinking water, teas or juices constantly will provide your body with adequate fluids which will work to thin out the secretions and make it easier to spit it out if needed.

Constipation

• Drink plenty of fluids unless restricted by your doctor.

• Increase fiber intake to 25-35 grams fiber/day by eating high fiber foods such as Grape Nuts, Shredded Wheat, oatmeal, quinoa, whole grain breads and pastas, beans and lentils.

• Take acacia fiber or psyllium husk powdered supplement. Discuss with your dietitian.

• Get moving! Literally, get up and walk, stretch, be active. This will help move those bowels.

• Prunes and dried apricots tend to work well in getting the bowels moving.

• ½ cup prune juice – some like to warm it up.

• Drink fennel tea.

• Consume yogurt daily for the live cultures which will normalize gut flora. May need to take a probiotic supplement daily. First try eating yogurt 1-3 times per day.

Diarrhea

• May try L-glutamine powder. L-glutamine (or just glutamine) is an amino acid that helps repair and heal the lining of the GI tract. Taking 15-30 grams/day for 2 weeks is a decent trial period. Always review use with your dietitian and/or doctor first.

Nurse's Note:

Pain medications can be very constipating. Drink plenty of water and take a stool softener suggested by your physician to help manage this side effect.

• To replace fluids and electrolytes (sodium and potassium) lost when you have diarrhea, drink water and electrolyte replacement drinks such as Gatorade and Powerade to name a couple of examples. Pedialyte would work also. Be sure to check with your doctor and nurse to make sure electrolyte drinks are not restricted for any reason.

• Have salty foods such as saltine crackers, broth and pretzels to replace sodium losses.

• Have foods high in potassium such as bananas, tomatoes, carrots, baked potato and plain yogurt to replace potassium losses.

• Increase soluble fiber in your diet such as applesauce, rice, bananas, and oatmeal. Acacia fiber powder is a soluble fiber that works to slowly regulate bowels.

• The only dairy foods you should have when experiencing diarrhea would be yogurt. It is recommended that yogurt be consumed 1-3 times daily to help normalize gut flora. If yogurt is not tolerated, you can take probiotic supplements in the amount of 7-15 billion live cells/day.

• Do not take vitamin C supplements when experiencing diarrhea.

Decreased Or No Appetite

• Try eating small amounts of food more often throughout the day. Make every bite count by choosing high calorie and protein foods such as nuts, seeds, soybeans (edamame), maybe make a trail mix with nuts and dried fruits and even bits of dark chocolate in there. Other suggestions include: hummus spread on carrots, yogurt with low fat granola, whole grain bread with nut butter, hard-boiled egg or cottage cheese and fruit.

• Take Omega-3s daily as they are anti-inflammatory and will help to counteract the inflammatory process that is making you a) not hungry and, b) when you are hungry you get full fast. I suggest 1500 mg Omega-3 fatty acids (EPA and DHA) daily. Do not take on an empty stomach, though. If you are not able to eat a lot, have a few crackers or half cup of soup before taking supplementation.

• Eat foods high in Omega-3s such as salmon, venison, buffalo, and walnuts, and use flaxseed and canola oils.

• Fruits, especially watermelon, are good to try when you are not feeling very hungry.

• Stay hydrated with water, flavored water, 100% juice popsicles, juices, rice water (congee) and broths.

• Smoothies, shakes and slushies are generally well-tolerated and you can pack in the calories by adding berries, fruits, carrots, milk, yogurt, protein powder, etc.

• You can drink a high calorie nutritional supplement. There are many to choose from and you can even make your own using whey or plant based protein powder. One calorie dense drink I do recommend to gain weight after a big weight loss or to prevent this from happening is Boost (formerly Carnation) VHC (Very High Calorie). This drink, unlike Ensure or regular Boost, is not available retail. You can ask at your cancer care facility or you can possibly contact a local home health company on your own and ask them if they carry this formula or something similar. A solid recommendation is to drink this throughout the day at a ¼ cup dose (equivalent to ¼ can), 4 times per day, refrigerating the formula in between drinks. This will equal one can total per day which is 560 calories. This can help to maintain weight, or at the very least minimize weight loss. What we don't want to happen is significant weight loss. This greatly affects your nutritional status and fighting power.

• An appetite stimulant may be necessary for a brief amount of time. There are a couple we most commonly use, Megace or Marinol. Discuss your appetite with your doctor, nurse and dietitian so that again, we can be proactive in managing your symptoms.

• Try yoga, stretching exercises, deep breathing, Guided Imagery with a licensed counselor, talking with someone or support group, or other means of relieving stress and anxiety that work for you.

Sore Throat/Painful And/Or Difficulty Swallowing

Sometimes radiation may cause some esophagitis. Try some of these tips to help minimize pain and troubles swallowing.

• Use Magic Mouthwash. It can numb area so that you can swallow.

• Consume mostly soft foods or liquids such as puddings, mashed potatoes, eggs, pasta, oatmeal or other desired hot cereals, protein shakes/smoothies/slushies, canned peaches or pears, yogurts, and cottage cheese.

• Drink milk (skim, soy, almond, or rice milk) between meals. If cancer is estrogenic, 1 cup per day soy milk is allowed.

• Sip soup and teas.

• Make frozen fruit sections (peaches, grapes cut in half, melons) and suck on them.

• There is something called capsaicin taffy. Capsaicin is a pain reliever and it is found in cayenne pepper. You can make it using a small amount of cayenne pepper. NEVER put cayenne pepper directly on your mouth or tongue as it is extremely spicy and hot.

CAPSAICIN TAFFY RECIPE:

1 cup sugar
¾ cup light corn syrup
2/3 cup water
1 tablespoon cornstarch
2 tablespoons soft margarine
1 teaspoon salt
2 teaspoons vanilla
½ to 1½ teaspoons cayenne pepper (powdered)

Begin by using only ½ teaspoon of the cayenne pepper in the first recipe you make and build up to 1½ teaspoons in following batches if it doesn't cause your mouth to burn. COMBINE: everything except vanilla and cayenne pepper cooking over medium heat stirring constantly, to 256 degrees Fahrenheit (use candy thermometer). Remove from heat and stir in vanilla and cayenne pepper. Once cooled enough to touch, pull taffy. Let cool on wax paper. When stiff, cut into strips, then pieces. Wrap in wax paper and store in cool, dry place.

Dry Mouth/Tender Mouth

• Sip water and teas frequently throughout the day to moisten mouth.

• Limit caffeine and alcohol intake as they tend to be a diuretic and pull fluid out of the body.

• Use a non-alcohol containing mouthwash such as Biotene. (big white bottle available at many local retail shops)

• Have water/water bottle with you at all times—take frequent sips.

• Consume moist foods such as stews, casseroles, soups, and fruits.

• Suck on ice chips, popsicles, or make slushies if cold temperature foods are desired and tolerated.

Nurse's Note:
If you use gum, mints, or hard candy to help with dry mouth, choose sugar free as sugar aids in the growth of yeast.

• Use broth, gravies, sauces, yogurt, silken tofu (moist and creamy), warm water, juices, milk or dairy alternatives, and coconut milk to moisten foods.

• Eat soft foods such as yogurt, all natural ice cream, oatmeal, pudding, Cream Of Wheat, Malt-O-Meal, even cooked vegetables such as cauliflower can be mashed to make "mock mashed potatoes".

• Use olive oil, canola oil, and/or coconut oil to make swallowing easier.

• Avoid crunchy textured foods, tough meats, and raw vegetables.

• Chew xylitol based gum. Xylitol is a sugar-free sweetener and does not promote tooth decay. This is available in most grocery stores down the "health food" or "all natural" sections of the store.

• Use a humidifier in your room at night to keep the air moist.

• Moisten lips frequently with lip balm, Aquafor, cocoa butter or olive oil.

Taste Changes

• Good oral hygiene is a must! Take good care of that mouth. A dry mouth can lead to increased bacteria growth so be sure to keep your mouth moistened and clean. If painful to brush, buy one of those sponge-ended toothbrushes and try using that for brushing.

• Mouthwash can make foods taste better. Rinse well prior to eating and see if this works for you. Biotene as an example of alcohol-free mouthwash that is typically better tolerated than those alcohol-containing mouthwashes.

• For metallic taste and dry mouth try sour food, if tolerated, such as lemon or lime in your drinking water which can work to increase saliva production, too. Eating fruits may also help to get rid of the bad taste.

• Try using plastic ware versus silverware if you have a metallic taste in your mouth.

• Cold foods such as chilled fruit, leaf salads, cold salads (egg, pasta, tuna or quinoa salads) are sometimes better tolerated if you are experiencing bitter or metallic taste changes as well as an "aftertaste".

• Try a variety of teas. Typically, mint teas do the trick to lessen bad taste changes.

• Zinc may help minimize or alleviate taste changes. Discuss zinc supplementation with your oncologist and dietitian.

• Marinate meats, chicken and fish in a sweet marinade— sweet and sour sauce, soy/ginger/honey mixture, or raspberry vinaigrette.

Nausea And Vomiting

• Consume colorless, odorless meals, especially before treatments. Research has shown that the meal you eat prior to treatment can make a difference in how likely you are to experience nausea and vomiting.

• If vomiting, it is most important to focus on keeping adequately hydrated as best you can. Sip fluids every 15 minutes at least. Try clear soda, sports drinks, Pedialyte, juices, popsicles, ice chips, ginger tea or other good-sounding tea, broth, ginger ale. If you are not able to keep things down for 24 – 48 hours, please call your nurse or case manager to let them know.

• Medications are available for nausea management. Discuss these with your oncologist and nurse.

Nurse's Note:

If vomiting is a problem during treatment, you may need to have IV fluids a few days a week to help support you during this critical time.

Nurse's Note:

If nausea is an issue, it may help to keep a food diary. This will help you decide which foods to eliminate during therapy to help alleviate side effects.

• Eat cold foods as they are generally better tolerated and tend to not trigger vomiting.

• Stick to the old standbys: crackers, dry toast, rice, oatmeal, grits or other hot cereal.

• You can try wearing Sea Bands around your wrist. They hit a trigger point and can help lessen feeling of nausea.

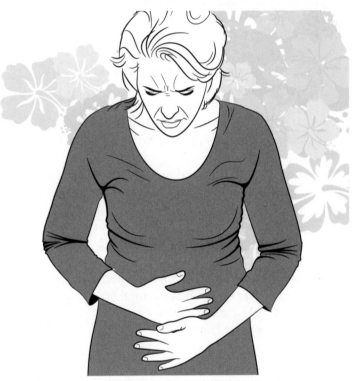

fig. 9.2

Let your providers know if you are experiencing nausea. With the many new medications available, nausea should not be a big issue for you.

Anemia

Anemia is when you do not have enough red blood cells. Red blood cells carry oxygen throughout your body and when you do not have enough you may feel tired, weak and/or short of breath. You doctor will be monitoring your lab work to watch for anemia. There are different types of anemia such as iron deficiency anemia or it can be due to low levels of B12 and folic acid. Sometimes anemia is caused by the cancer itself. For iron deficiency anemia, an iron supplement may be ordered by the doctor. It is best to go with a non-constipating iron such as ferrous bis-glycinate. Also try eating high iron foods such as meats, chicken, turkey, or fish. These are called heme sources meaning they come from the blood of the animal. There are non-heme sources like beans, lentils and green leafies. When eating these non-heme sources, have vitamin C with it to increase absorption.

fig. 9.3

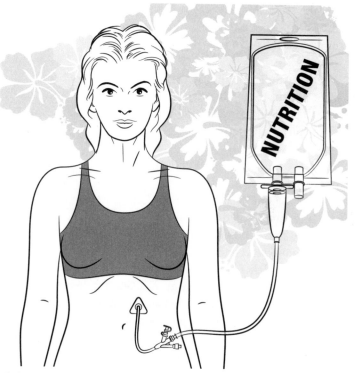

NUTRITION

A feeding tube can become a "life-line" for you during cancer treatment if excessive weight loss is a problem.

Weight Loss/Gain

During treatment it may become increasing difficult to manage weight. If having difficulty maintaining weight, continue attempts at eating and drinking as much as possible.

Nurse's Note:

Your nurse will weigh you at least weekly during treatment. This may occur more often if weight loss is a concern.

As mentioned before, this can be done with sips of water and caloric liquids such as juices, popsicles, smoothies, protein shakes or slushies, etc. If being treated with radiation and/or chemo, esophagitis may occur if it is in the field of radiation making it difficult to eat and drink adequate calories. Do not be alarmed, but a feeding tube may be needed temporarily as a means of nourishing your body until your whole GI tract can be used. It's plain and simple, if you can't swallow your food/liquids, you can't meet your nutritional needs. If part of your GI tract is not working properly, nutrition support may be needed. Just know all attempts to help you nourish your body the old fashioned way will be upheld. Be proactive and tell your doctor about any difficulties you may have in maintaining a healthy weight during treatment.

Weight gain is a common complaint made by a breast cancer patient to the dietitian. Weight gain is seen most likely due to a combination of being thrust into menopause and being less physically active.

SUPPLEMENTS

The AICR (American Institute of Cancer Research) has made a recommendation to take minimal supplements while increasing nutrient density of your food intake. We do know from recent research that many of us are deficient in vitamin D. Vitamin D deficiencies are linked with cancer, MS, depression, insomnia, aches/pains, etc. Getting your vitamin D tested is highly recommended and from there it can be determined if vitamin D3 supplementation is necessary. A decent maintenance dose is 1000 IU/day, doubling that in the winter months to 2000 IU/day. Testing is necessary to follow up on vitamin D levels to assure there is no toxicity, as well as to be sure adequate amounts of vitamin D3 is taken.

Nurse's Note:

Ask your doctor or nurse about nutrition supplements.

Fish oil, as mentioned, is often recommended because of its anti-inflammatory properties. 1500-3000 mg/day Omega-3s is recommended each day. The Omega-3s are DHA and EPA. Look for the content of these on the back of the supplement bottle. Add up the DHA and EPA to equal the recommended daily dose. Concentrations vary greatly so be sure to take adequate amounts. Carlson brand name offers a quality Omega-3 product. If scheduled to have surgery, be sure to tell your surgeon and all physicians involved you are taking fish oil. It is recommended that fish oil be stopped prior to procedures as it thins out the blood.

A multivitamin a day is usually appropriate. Go over contents of it with your registered dietitian and/or doctor. A "clean" product is the best, meaning there are no fillers, preservatives, and maybe even hypo-allergenic, using no wheat, soy or derivatives. Some suggestions are Metagenics, Thorne, and Nordic Naturals. These companies offer clean products as do many others. They are only available through a health professional.

A fiber supplement such as acacia fiber, is beneficial if you are prone to constipation or extreme cycles of diarrhea then constipation. If you have increased fiber in your diet by incorporating whole grains, fruits and vegetables, supplementation may not be necessary.

The great debate continues on whether to take antioxidant supplementation during treatment or not. Healthcare practitioners vary greatly on their stance regarding what is allowed or not allowed during treatment and you will need to discuss this with your oncologist. Listen to your body. You have a mind/body connection and need to listen to it. If you feel confident that something is working for you, do it, as long as treatment is not compromised in any way. Don't do some supplement just because someone told you about it and it worked for them or because of what you read on the internet. You will get tons of advice at every turn, but take time to digest it all and figure out what works for you. Rather than focusing on supplementation for added nutrients, it is better to focus on maximizing your nutrient intake through food.

You can go to **www.ORACvalues.com**. ORAC stands for oxygen radical absorbance capacity, which is the antioxidant power of foods. **ORACvalues.com** is a comprehensive database of foods and offers a list of determined antioxidant levels. Some things high in ORAC are: parsley, blueberries and cinnamon. Check out the website to see what others are high in ORAC values! NOTE: *Always discuss all meds, natural supplements, vitamins and minerals with your doctor to assure nothing is compromising your treatment.*

Recommended Books:

Eating Well Through Cancer – distributed by Merck

The Cancer Lifeline Cookbook – by Kimberly Mathai MS, RD, with Ginny Smith

The Cancer-Fighting Kitchen and One Bite at a Time – by Rebecca Katz

In the above-mentioned books you will find whole-foods based recipes and wonderfully helpful nutrition information.

Online Resources:

The world of online information is vast. "Googling" has become a way of life but be careful in what sites you go to. There is one theory found online that gets brought up the most. It is the theory that "sugar feeds cancer". Please remember one thing: anything growing inside of us will be fueled by what we are fueled by. Our main energy source is glucose. This is sugar. As stated before, follow the 80/20 rule of thumb with regards to diet and nutrition. Most definitely do not avoid fruits and whole grains in hopes of depriving your body of sugar or in hopes of starving the tumor. Keep the focus on balance of carbohydrates, proteins, and good fats. Eat whole grains, bright or dark colored produce, plant proteins, lean or lower fat animal proteins, and good fats.

Recommended Websites:

There are numerous websites to view. So much so it can be overwhelming. Here is a list of credible websites:

www.caring4cancer.com/go/cancer/nutrition - side effects mgmt-written by registered dietitian.

www.cancer.org

www.cancerrd.com

www.cancer.gov

www.nlm.nih.gov/medlineplus

www.aicr.org/site/PageServer

www.mypyramidtracker.gov/planner/

www.oralcancerfoundation.org/dental/xerostomia.htm - information on dry mouth.

www.foodnews.org – for the Dirty Dozen annual report on produce.

www.consumerlabs.com – to review your supplement. See if it passed quality testing.

www.ORACvalues.com – to review antioxidant levels of foods.

www.livestrong.org

www.asha.org/public/speech/disorders/SwallowingProbs.htm - American Speech Language and Hearing Institute.

Part Ten

Calming The Emotional Storm Of Breast Cancer

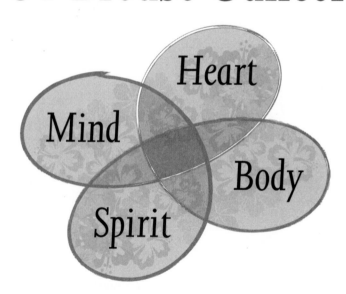

Calming The Emotional Storm

A diagnosis of breast cancer is a crisis large enough to impact your body, your mind, your heart, and your spirit. Breast cancer is a family disease because it affects everyone you love, and in different ways. Today women and men with breast cancer are living longer and healthier lives than ever before. Even so, it remains a large enough crisis to change your life immediately in ways that cause you to suffer, and in other more positive ways you won't recognize until later, perhaps much later. You have a lot of work ahead as you face treatment and living with a chronic disease, as breast cancer is understood today. You will feel discouraged and then find your strength and resilience over and over. If you think about it, curing and healing are different. The work of your physicians is to find a cure, or ways to prolong your life. You have an equally important job. Your job is to find ways and people who can help you heal the emotional and spiritual suffering generated by breast cancer, and to allow cancer to become your teacher. To be able to manage your new and different life you must learn to truly live, grow, express your own needs, and have your own back.

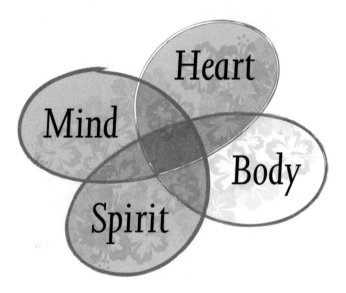

Breast Cancer And Your Body:
Your Physical Experience

"Why does the smallest part of me give me the most trouble?!"

"I blamed myself for this. Nobody in my family has had it. I

thought I got this because I didn't take good care of my body. I never learned how to manage my stress. I finally stopped hating myself when my doctor asked me this: 'Where do you want your focus to be—on blaming yourself or on healing?' I had to choose, since I couldn't focus on both. I chose healing."

"I bought some beautiful camisoles. I need to hide from his eyes for awhile."

"I feel guilty. I've worked since I was 16. The rest of society is working. Am I being lazy taking time off for treatment?"

"You'll hear me say 'I haven't got the energy'. But please keep asking me anyway."

"It takes a lot to preserve my dignity and my sense of myself now. I'm tired all of the time."

"I had no idea what the cost of this journey would be when I started treatment. I'd still do it, and fight to live, but I couldn't understand at the beginning."

"I wish I'd had more information about the side effects of radiation before I had them. Maybe somebody told me, but I was surprised and scared. I needed them written out in real language, not medicalese."

"I have friends who have had breast cancer. They smile and assure me I can do the treatment, all of it. They are so encouraging. I don't know what I'd do without them."

"Is this the best I'm going to feel? I might be taking treatment for years. I can't do what I used to do, like hike in the mountains. If this is as good as it's going to get, what makes my life worth living?"

Tips For The Journey:

Remember that your whole body is not sick, although it may feel like that. Aside from the cancer, how well is your

Nurse's Note:

Don't hesitate to let your caregivers know how you are feeling. They are there to help you.

body working for you now? Some people feel more hopeful when they remember that, in general, their body is doing well, in spite of the cancer.

Think about all the ways your body has stood by you in the past, the times you've been ill and recovered, the times your body has responded well to medical interventions, the ways your body has told you what it needs and how you have responded. You're simply doing that again, even with the cancer. Your body knows how to heal.

Respect the needs of your body as you move through treatment. Many people with breast cancer feel exhausted by treatment. You will need more rest than you think. Don't push your body, which is working so hard to absorb and process different medications and procedures while maintaining normal functioning at the same time. Your body is working overtime to get you well again and to heal, which requires enormous energy. Lovingly, give it a break.

It's important to bring someone with you to doctor appointments and chemo sessions. This needs to be someone you don't have to take care of, or entertain, or even talk to. Choose someone who can just sit and be with you, who can be another listening ear when your medical team gives you information. Research shows that people hear about 20% of the information presented to them when they are stressed, not to mention when chemo brain (the temporary, short term memory loss associated with chemotherapy) complicates memory and communication.

Nurse's Note:

Make sure you have a friend or family member with you for medical appointments to help take notes.

After surgery, husbands or partners can feel pressured to tell you that you look fine, when they may not initially feel that way. If you are heading into surgery, close your eyes for a moment and imagine surgery is complete and has gone very well, and the bandages are being removed. With your mind's eye, look down where your breast was and imagine what you see. What is your very first reaction? Can you give your husband or partner the gift of the same first reaction you imagine yourself feeling?

Whether or not you decide to have reconstructive surgery done, you will experience a period of time when you are adjusting to your new appearance. Many women have ambivalent feelings about the surgery; they are grateful to be alive, to have the obvious cancer removed, but dislike how they look or feel. This can be especially true for women whose breasts are a crucial part of their sexuality or key to feeling like a woman. Allow yourself to take the time you need to come to terms privately with your "new" breast or breasts. Allow yourself to grieve. Talk about your feelings with your partner. Women often assume the change will be very upsetting to their partners, when in fact they will come to terms with the loss just as you will. A breast cancer support group can be a big help at this time, since women who have been in the group for awhile are often comfortable showing newcomers their own reconstructed breasts. Having no reconstruction is also an option many women are most comfortable with. Some women like their reconstructed breasts better than the originals. Over time you will come to terms with your new look, and gratitude for health will outweigh your doubts about how your breasts look or feel.

Prioritize the precious energy you have. Decide what you want to do, then pace yourself so that you can avoid "crashing" into exhaustion and the misery that comes with it. Is completing a task most important, so that you can feel useful? Is it sharing time with a loved one that will fill your need today? Make a list of what you'd like to do. Choose. You probably can't do everything on your list, so trim it in order to stay focused on what you can do, instead of what you can't. If you choose to do more than your level of energy can handle, schedule time to rest so your body can get back to healing. You'll feel more in control and content.

Ask the people who love you for some ideas of things you can do that don't require physical effort. If chemo brain is holding you captive, ask for ideas for movies you might like. Funny movies are good for your immune system. War-like films might inspire the fight in you. Books with short stories or stories of how others with cancer have coped, healed or

Nurse's Note:

Some people like to journal during treatment. This helps clarify and express their feelings.

Nurse's Note:

Talk to others who have been through the same or similar treatments. Don't hesitate to ask them questions.

gained wisdom can help. Meet your own needs.

Allow people to help you. Be specific in your requests. People with cancer say that it's much harder to receive than to give, but remember: you are giving people a gift by receiving their help. They feel helpless, and any ways they are allowed to be helpful to you helps them, too. They're a part of your team. Relinquish thoughts that you can handle this journey alone, or that your family can manage it alone. When friends ask what they can do to help, ask one of them to organize a work party for you. Have a good friend make up the work list. Your job is to join them by doing the least demanding job on the list, or to sit back and rest, feeling loved and cared for.

The goal is not to endure stress, but to manage it. Receiving help is a management skill.

Reduce the physical challenges of treatment by finding ways to help yourself relax. Feeling the need to be constantly alert, ready for battle, sword in hand, is common among people facing a life-threatening disease. It can help prevent more bad news from being the kind of shock you felt at your first diagnosis. But the need to relax during your cancer journey is crucial for your healing, and the price of remaining hyper-vigilant is always feeling the threat of more cancer hanging over your head. Letting go for awhile with a hot bath, yoga, relaxation exercises, guided imagery, massage, meditation or prayer will help strengthen your immune system, your mood, and your ability to bring new energy to the fight.

Perhaps most important of all, remember that you are not the disease. You are not the problem. Cancer is. You are much more than the cancer. You are a person who is loved and valued, well or sick, vital or exhausted.

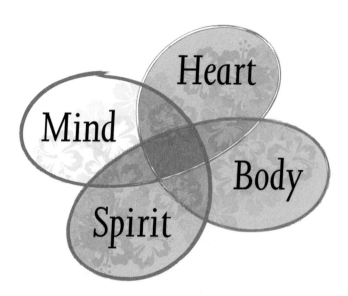

Mind Heart Body Spirit

Breast Cancer And Your Mind:
Your Thoughts And Beliefs About Cancer

"My doctor said something that really helped. He said 'Don't pay any attention to statistics or anecdotal information. It's your cancer, not anybody else's.'"

"Cancer is not my diagnosis—it's our diagnosis. I want to protect my whole family from being scared, but it's really hard to protect them from my fears and communicate well at the same time. I keep biting my tongue."

"I heard the word cancer and I didn't hear another thing. I feel like I can't even think. All I can do is feel, and feel scared."

"I'm terrified most of the time. I try not to listen to everything people say so I can stay focused on today and the next step I have to take."

"Some of my friends can't come with me into my cancer world. They keep talking about my reconstructive surgery when I'll be 'back to normal again'. But I'll never be the same person I used to be. What if they don't like me then? What if I don't feel close to them?"

"The life I knew is gone. It's over. My goal was to get to 70 years old without taking any meds. I was an icon of health. I have to learn to think differently about my health now."

"Everybody has ideas of what I should do and how I should handle this, and I don't know who to listen to."

"I'm the 'caregiver' I read about. I'm her husband. She's always asked how she's doing. People don't ask me that. Why not? I'm overwhelmed."

She: "I don't talk about pain. I don't want to explain it all the time. I don't care about the broken dishwasher!"

He: "When she's in pain or tired she's short tempered, grumpy and she barks at me. I need to not take it personally."

"I have to ask people to help me. That's easier to do now that I'm not so angry at the world for my getting cancer."

"I just deny that I could die. I don't even think about it. Is something wrong with me?"

"I had to change my whole perception of my cancer. I finally allowed myself to be ill. I accepted my illness, and then I could let go of so much suffering."

"I'm the key member of my medical team here. I'm the key decision maker."

"Go ahead and change doctors if you don't feel you 'click' with the doctor you have, or if you're not getting your questions answered. Do you wonder what chemo is like? Or radiation? Ask! This is your life you're fighting for!"

"The scheduler told me 'We can't get you in for two weeks' and I freaked. I wanted to yell 'Don't you understand? I'm dying of cancer here!' That was 4 years ago. I'm so thankful that urgency is gone."

"I feel limited by my own thinking. I don't want to plan things. If I leave town and something goes wrong, what would I do?"

"I'm done with treatment. Am I done with cancer? How can I stay well by myself?"

"I felt the need to do the paperwork—you know, the end of life decisions—so that when I die nobody has to deal with all of that. My family was horrified that I found it comforting."

"I was the rock in the family. I knew what everyone should do and how to do it. I can't do that any more. They need to be their own rock and use their own best judgment from now on."

Tips For The Journey:

For many there is an urge to stay silent in order to protect loved ones from powerful fears and anger, and an equally strong need to talk. Find someone you can be totally honest with, who can listen without giving advice or opinions. Allow yourself to express your fears fully so that you can let them go for now. This might be someone in your family or it might be a trusted friend. You can contact a cancer support group in your area. These are the people who really get it, since they are dealing with some of the same issues themselves. You can seek the loving ear of a spiritual advisor or a psychotherapist. Be wary of internet chat rooms and blogs. Many people become more frightened while exploring because they are exposed to other peoples' fears.

Just as you need the freedom and space to express your feelings, so do your children or grandchildren. Your cancer center may offer (or be willing to start) a national project of the Annie E. Casey Foundation called Kidz Count, which welcomes children whose parent or grandparent has cancer. Without this program, many children feel alone and unable to find the words or support from peers to help with the feelings that haunt them.

Nurse's Note:

It is important for you to be comfortable with your care team. This is just as important to them as it is to you.

Many couples, when one partner is diagnosed with cancer, try to protect the other from their deep fears and concerns, and choose not to talk about how they are really doing. This can cause an invisible wall to descend between you, making you feel like friendly roommates instead of intimate partners. It can become harder and harder to talk honestly when this happens. Some people find themselves having the most personal conversations only with someone other than their partner, which, over time, can cause damage to the relationship. Go ahead and cry together, talk together, listen to each other's fears, and comfort each other. Get some couples counseling if you need it; this is a time of crisis. You'll feel less alone and you'll know that you're part of a team facing the cancer together. This, over time, will strengthen your relationship. Join a cancer support group together or look for a caregiver support group in your area so your spouse or partner can get help with feelings of isolation, frustration, fear and guilt so common to these special people whose world has turned upside down as well. Many religious organizations, the Quakers and Mormons among them, form a "care committee" to organize help when anyone among them is sick or disabled. You can do this, too.

Couples can find it helpful to talk about their relationship when one of them becomes ill. Every couple has made agreements, spoken and unspoken, about how they will be with each other. A wedding vow is such a contract. It can be helpful to clarify the unspoken assumptions you each hold about illness, what caring for each other means during illness, and what it means to give and receive support.

Be aware that some of your friends may appear to withdraw from you when they discover you have cancer. You may be thinking, "When you get cancer you sure find out who your friends are." The truth is that they don't know what to say to you, or they are afraid they will cry in your presence, adding the burden of their fears or grief to your load. The longer this estrangement goes on, the guiltier they feel. Instead of feeling abandoned you could choose to initiate contact with them and let them know you miss them and would welcome their presence, in a real way, at this time.

On the other hand, there may be friends who you'd rather not be in contact with now. When you're with them you may feel their needs weighing you down, or that you need to use precious energy to attend to them. You may simply want to avoid the ubiquitous question, "How ARE you?", asked with deep concern. An option is to go online to sites such as Caring Bridge or Helping Hands, where you can enter information and updates you're comfortable sharing that others can access. This will give you more privacy and prevent you from having to answer the same questions over and over. Friends and acquaintances can send you messages this way, too.

Most people fighting cancer hear intense and heartfelt advice about which doctors to see and which alternative or complementary treatments to try. Some can be very insistent. This can be very confusing and frightening. If this kind of talk is not helpful, you can respond by saying, "Thanks for your thoughts and for caring about me, but I trust the doctors I'm working with and I'm not looking for other treatments right now. I'll let you know if I change my mind." If you are interested in finding an oncology naturopath to complement your medical treatment, look online. You may be able to consult on the phone if the doctor is located at a distance. Most important of all, trust the carefully considered decisions you, your loved ones and your doctors have chosen to help you heal.

Sometimes people say they're coping by being in denial. They are simply pacing themselves, accepting information at a speed they can tolerate as time goes by. From diagnosis through treatment, cancer is a long haul.

People with cancer are often approached by friends and co-workers who, for some reason, feel free to share the most horrifying, tragic stories of cancer suffering they know. Be prepared. You'll hear stories about relatives, friends, friends of friends, and strangers and all of the ways they suffered. Allow yourself to immediately interrupt these stories, saying something like, "That story makes me feel nervous, uncomfortable, bad, or _____. Let's talk about something else."

When treatment is done a new set of challenges appear. There is no going "back to normal". There is only moving forward, creating a "new normal" life. You will find yourself relaxing into your new life if you take the time to deeply consider what you've been left with after cancer, what you've been gifted with by the cancer, what you choose to bring into your life now, and what you choose to leave behind. One thing that stays is this: you will wonder if cancer will come back and kill you until you die of something else. You can make this decision: "If I have to deal with cancer again, I will."

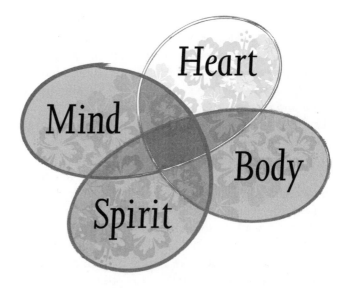

Breast Cancer And Your Heart:
The Ways You Feel About Yourself, Your Life, And Cancer

"I'm so scared all the time. I've heard so many awful things about treatment. Poison, slash and burn. How will I survive this? Some days all I want to do is walk away from it all."

"I got the shovel out again today. I'm digging my own grave. I've got to get a handle on my anxiety."

"My three year old saw a bald mannequin in a store and yelled 'Look Mommy! She's bald, just like you!' I can't hide my cancer, even with this great wig."

"I hate my body. I hate how it feels. I hate the scars. I hate my breast being gone. My whole body is way off. It's not me."

"Why don't I feel anything? What's wrong with me?"

"I know I have to keep a positive attitude or I'll die."

"If my test comes back bad, I'm screwed. If it comes back with good news, I still worry."

"I have anxiety, but I'm slowing my pace as I race to the edge of the cliff. My life doesn't feel like it's going to explode the way it did when I got diagnosed. Everything I worry about doesn't need to be weighed so heavily. I'm finding my balance."

"I feel so useless when I don't have any energy. I always took charge. I was the one people depended on. I just can't be that person now. I feel like such a burden on my family."

"I get so scared about my medical care sometimes. If I'm unhappy with something they say or do, and I'm not nice, will they give up on me or not try so hard to save my life? I finally asked my doctor that and she was amazed. She wanted to know when I wasn't happy. So make sure you ask your questions, and insist on answers in ways you understand. It will give you a sense of control."

"How will my having no breasts affect my husband in the long run? Now he's OK with it, but what about 5 years from now? Will he want to have an affair?"

"I thought my husband wasn't attracted to me during treatment, but it was me that I wasn't attracted to."

"I'm done tormenting myself about how I look now. I'm done."

"When my wife was diagnosed, my first thought was 'Everybody knows it's a death sentence. She's going to die.' For the first six months there was so much fear and anger. My brain was consumed with thoughts of cancer and treatment and survival. Now, four and a half years into it, here we are, happier than we've ever been. I'm not raging at the world. Our focus is on today, on right now. We watch birds eating mountain ash berries. Did you know some birds eat them whole and others eat only the insides?"

"I'm finally mad about what cancer has done to the life I had."

"I'm beginning to understand that I deserve all the help I'm getting. It's a big step from feeling desperate, like I had to have it but was putting everyone out. I deserve it. Isn't that amazing?"

"I'm a man with breast cancer. Try telling that to your friends. It's embarrassing. I don't want to talk about it."

"My family and friends can get a break from the cancer by withdrawing from me for awhile. I can never get a break."

"I just can't bring myself to discipline the kids any more. In case I die, I don't want to leave them with bad memories. It drives my husband crazy."

"I do the cancer stomp dance with my kids when any of us gets scared. We laugh. It helps."

"If I relax and put the fear down, the cancer will sneak up on me again. I never want to feel that shock of being diagnosed with cancer again."

"When I'm depressed I go somewhere else. I stop. I freeze in place and quit taking care of myself."

"I don't feel whole any more. I want the lives my friends are living."

"Losing my hair felt like one more insult. My cancer became public. I was so embarrassed. I had to become willing to just let myself be embarrassed, but in a softer way. It's not my fault this happened."

"Sex? What's that?"

"Is it depression or is it grief? I think it's grief. I've lost so much."

"What's the hardest loss for me, even though I've been told there's no more evidence of cancer? I'll always wonder if it will come back and kill me. I've lost forever the assumption that I'll die of old age."

"I was sexually assaulted when I was younger. I look at where my breast used to be and feel the way I felt then all over again. I feel like the abuse will never end."

"I long for the carefree days I didn't even know were carefree."

"I'm done with treatment. When am I going to feel like 'YIPPEE! I DID IT!'?"

"I'm done with treatment. I actually feel good. My husband and family are absolutely convinced I'm fine again. They can't grieve with me. I don't think I'll ever be done with cancer. I'm in a new world again and I don't understand this one, either."

"Breast cancer is so life changing. Now that treatment is done it's still life changing because I don't know how to really live without the routines of treatment, which were so reassuring. My hand was held all the way along. Smart people really had me covered. Now where am I? Who am I? I feel alone with my fears that it will come back. I've made the tamoxifen my routine now, my big morning ritual. My husband thinks I'm nuts."

"Since treatment I'm realizing that we can help our bodies, but we really can't control them. I can hold this truth now without so much pain. It's just life. It moves on. It's all OK, in the long run."

"I wouldn't trade what I've learned from cancer for anything. I was always running in my life. I'm sitting in my life now. I've learned how to replace the old, constant judgment with compassion and respect for myself. That is the gift cancer gave to me. Or maybe I gave it to myself."

"In nature time is so different. It slows down. Don't tie time to a clock. Who knows how long any of us will live?"

"I have regrets. I have not lived my life very fully. I've made compromises I wish I hadn't, trying to meet other people's expectations. Cancer changed that. I'm a lot happier with myself now."

"I want to leave a legacy of good work. I may need to leave my work unfinished, unresolved. That breaks my heart."

"When I was first diagnosed I was so stressed I felt close to suicide. I didn't want to hurt anybody, but I just wanted to feel some peace. Then, after a couple of treatments I thought 'OK, I can do this.' I felt much more relaxed. Now, after several years, I don't think about cancer. I think instead about each day. I focus on one day, one symptom at a time."

"I'm learning to check inside and ask myself 'What is the truth here and what is the fear?' I try to separate them now."

"Imagining dying is easier than imagining being happy again."

He: "It's not about her dying somewhere down the road. It's about loving her now. Worrying about her dying is wasting precious time. To people just hearing they have breast cancer, or any cancer, I'd say 'You will get to a place where you know this and are more at peace. I promise.'"

Tips For The Journey:

It will help if you think back on the hardest times you have already survived in your life. How did you make it through? What coping skills did you depend on? Did you need to talk, or withdraw for awhile? Did you allow yourself to feel sad, or angry? Did gathering information help? Did you need to turn the whole thing over to the "professionals" to "fix" so that you could relax? Did you have ways to distract yourself when you needed that? Did you pray? Did you allow people who loved you to help you? How? What worked back then? Tell a trusted friend the stories of how life has taught you these skills.

Think about the strengths of character you bring to this challenge. Recognize your wisdom, your inner power, your determination. What qualities did you bring to the critical times you've already survived in your life? If you're not sure, ask people who love you. They often see us more clearly than we see ourselves, especially when we are anxious. And, again, tell the stories of how life taught you to find these strengths within yourself.

There is a difference between grief and depression. When we grieve we know exactly why we feel so low. When we are depressed we often live in a cloud of unease and sadness without really knowing why. Sometimes people feel both. Things that used to bring you pleasure, or even deep joy, may feel empty now. Grieve through the losses that diagnosis and treatment have forced upon you. Meetings with a counselor can help you figure out where you are stuck, ways that might help you feel more centered and peaceful, and whether an anti-depressant would help for the time being.

Conflict often happens in families when differing ways of coping with the cancer collide. It is important to allow people to cope in their own ways. For example, one person may be devastated by fears that you will die. Another may be totally focused on what you need to do to complete treatment. Or, one person, in order to relax, may need to hear every update, attend all of your doctor appointments and treatment sessions. For others, this might cause unbearable stress. The statements to avoid among family members are: "You shouldn't feel that way" and, "If you love ___ (the person with cancer) enough you'd ___."

Men and women can have different ways of feeling and coping with breast cancer. Men often feel helpless because they can't fix the women they love, and work hard to get life back to "normal" as quickly as possible. Women can feel as though he doesn't understand or welcome their need to express fear, sadness and anger. It helps if women can find a breast cancer support group and close friends who can listen. It helps the relationship if both partners can understand and accept that men may not always be able to accompany their partners on the emotional journey of breast cancer.

It is normal to feel very frightened when breast cancer is diagnosed. It is also normal for emotions to sink below awareness at diagnosis. In a crisis we must stay focused. However, don't be surprised later when the feelings of crisis have passed (which they will) and your feelings from diagnosis rise to the surface. If this happens, remember that your emotions are simply catching up with the rest of you. Let yourself express them with someone you trust who can simply listen without having to "fix" you.

Remember this: you are not the burden weighing on the people who love you. The cancer is burdening all of you. For every family, when cancer is diagnosed, the fear of death is real, painful, and lasting. This is called anticipatory grief and it happens when any loved one's life is threatened, whether they die from the disease or not. That is part of the burden cancer places on all of you. Ask someone close to you to remind you of this, that you are not the burden, when you forget it. Most people do.

Children around the age of five (and older) always wonder if their parent is going to die from the cancer. Many of them will come right out and ask, while others hold this secret dread deep inside, causing physical symptoms or fears of going to school and leaving you alone at home. Children also wonder if they caused your cancer. This is what your children need from you: to know that they are loved and will be cared for by someone they trust during those times when you can't. They need to continue their normal routines such as music lessons and sports practices and games. The family rules, like bedtimes, time spent on computer games, etc., need to be maintained as closely as possible. Your children need to hear these promises from you: "I promise that the cancer is not your fault. I promise that I will tell you if I'm going to die from the cancer. Dying is not something the doctors are worried about at all now. So you don't need to worry about it. I want you to promise in exchange that you will come and talk with me when you are scared about this or anything else. I want to hear from you about anything else you want to talk to me about, too."

Learn to receive. Many people find this to be embarrassing, and question whether they deserve what their loved ones want to give. How can we learn to receive? Sometimes cancer forces the issue. For example, when you just cannot do the things necessary for your own well being, you have to ask for help. Other times, you can ease into it, intentionally receiving a bit, then more (like having a friend take your children to soccer practices). Ask yourself: would your loved ones deserve to receive help and care from you, were your circumstances reversed? Then why not you? Consider this: how would you feel if they refused your offer of help? Cancer, thankfully, has a way of severely disrupting the perfectionist standards many of us learned in childhood.

Depend on your loved ones. They want you to. Let them know what you'd like them to do for you. You could even ask them to do something you would do if you could for someone else. One woman had her sister tell their mother about the recurrence so that she would not have to see the look on her mother's face. That way she didn't have to bear the full load of disclosing the bad news. Avoid expressing your gratitude constantly, in a guilty way. Let yourself receive. One

Nurse's Note:

Learning how to deal with stress can help you maintain a healthier immune system to help you heal.

127

heartfelt thank you is enough.

One of the ways people stay balanced while living with cancer is to imagine their hands held open before them, one holding the reality "I might live. I just might live." The other hand holds the reality "This cancer might take my life long before I ever thought I'd die." Those who grasp only the possibility of living can become very anxious, for the opposite reality is also possible. Those who grasp only the possibility of dying sooner than they hoped can become stuck in depression. Hold both possibilities, lightly if you can, and remember: the weights in your hands will fluctuate, back and forth. The days you feel dispirited and down won't last. The days you feel filled with hope and confident you'll do well won't either. Remember the cancer motto: "Right now I'm OK. If that changes I'll deal with it, because that's what I do."

Consider joining a cancer support group. Although you are unique in your experience of cancer, the other group members are the only people who can come close to really understanding how you feel. Many cancer centers provide support for caregivers, too.

If you're not drawn to a support group, you can ask one of your medical providers, like your oncologist, a nurse, or the oncology counselor to contact another person with breast cancer and ask if he or she would be willing to contact you. Many people going through or finishing treatment themselves volunteer to call others who could use a listening ear. These relationships can become special and powerful sources of support, encouragement, and understanding.

Consider starting a fear journal that you write in for only 15-20 minutes at a time, perhaps daily, or when you feel the need. Pour your fears into it and then close it, leaving them there. Don't read and re-read it. Let them stay there. You might also start a list of things you'd like to do for the next week, month, or the next year. These aren't plans, but hopes. Planning for only a short time ahead can remind you of living well in spite of cancer and prevent you from feeling overwhelmed or uncomfortable.

Having cancer is a lonely experience. You probably feel alone, even if you are embraced by an entire group of people who love you, added to an excellent team of medical professionals, along with even the prayers of strangers. This is a time when you will learn to love and care for yourself in new ways. You will find strengths and resilience, paths to peace and rest, because cancer will teach you these things. This you can trust.

If you are a woman who has struggled with sexual abuse or assault in the past, it is normal to feel those feelings all over again when you endure the invasive experience of treatment for breast cancer. If you have not already done so, seek a counselor who can help you manage your feelings, supporting and guiding you toward the deep wisdom and acceptance that working through such hurts can generate. This process of supported healing can help you come to terms with the losses caused by assault so that you can think of them without the hurt and difficult feelings that you have lived with for so long. A kind, loving, and skilled therapist who can help you with emotional exploration and expression will provide the most effective assistance. If you are in crisis, a therapist also trained in EFT (Emotional Freedom Technique) or EMDR (Eye Movement Desensitization and Reprocessing), can help you learn to calm your anxious feelings quickly.

If you are a man with breast cancer, as 1% of breast cancer survivors are, you may carry the added burden of embarrassment at having what many consider to be a woman's disease. You may not be welcome at women's breast cancer support groups where a lot of "show and tell" happens. However, your needs for support are just as important. The cancer center may offer a general cancer support group you could attend. People there will understand and have your back.

Feeling embarrassed about hair loss or looking as exhausted as you feel can be very hard. When friends ask if there is something they can do for you, you might suggest they take you to buy a beautiful scarf or take you to consult with a make-up specialist. You could suggest a scarf party be held for you. Have the organizer suggest people buy only soft, cotton scarves for you, since they won't slip on your head when your hair is gone. You may feel more at peace with your appearance if you surrender to it and find ways to kindly see yourself through the long walk of hair re-growth and energy renewal, replacing critical self-talk with kindness and acceptance, in soft and loving tones.

Sexuality. So many women struggling with side effects from treatment are upset about the sudden and what feels like permanent, irrevocable disappearance of their sexual feelings. Feelings of guilt can exist for both partners, one for not wanting to make love, the other for wanting to. Talk together about ways that are comfortable and meaningful to physically express your love. The spontaneity of love-making can feel lost, but remember when you first began your sexual relationship? For many, there was nothing spontaneous about it. You spent time and effort preparing, lighting candles, choosing what to wear, selecting special music. When cancer treatment is done, your sexual feelings may well return, and for many couples, getting through such a crisis together has strengthened their relationship so that love making becomes an even deeper, more loving experience than it was before.

Beware of something that might called "the positive trap". No doubt you have heard the well-meaning advice, "Be positive!", many times, in many ways. People with cancer fear that if they are not thinking positively they will not get well, and might even die. But the opposite is true. Research shows that holding in the "negative" feelings such as anxiety, anger or sadness can be harmful to immune function in an indirect way. Expression of emotions—all of them—is an important part of staying healthy throughout the cancer journey. It is important to know someone who can listen to all of your emotions, hopeful and not, without imparting judgment or fear. By expressing them, you can let the scary feelings go and learn to take one day, or even one moment, at a time. Remember this cancer motto: "In this moment I am OK. If that changes I'll deal with it, because that's what I do". Tape this to a place where you will see it every day. Remember it. It's true.

People express emotions in a variety of ways. You may need to cry or you may feel relieved simply to acknowledge or describe your feelings of sadness. Men and women are often different in this way. No one way is better than another.

There are other benefits of expressing your fears, anger and sadness with someone you trust. When you do, hope that was hidden under those feelings bubbles up to the surface of your awareness. Expressing fears frees the hope to rise.

Sometimes people with cancer feel their hopes have died. Hopes that cannot be realized die, but new hopes always wait in the wings for us to discover them. What are you hoping for today? Make a list of your hopes, the ones that will make today better, and the big ones you hope to be fulfilled down the road. Review your list frequently, revise it, and share it with someone you're close to. This can lighten your spirit, and help define what you choose to do with the energy you have to use today.

When you become most discouraged, call a meeting with your closest friends and ask them to tell you why they want you to live. Allow their words to sink into you, encourage you, give you comfort, and inspire you.

Consider asking your care team for a referral to an oncology family therapist or counselor who can see you individually or include your family and other loved ones. Such a person can explore ways of coping that will work for you and help you all manage the many, sometimes conflicting ways people cope with their fear of losing someone they love and depend upon.

As we have seen, an experience of cancer changes people and the lives they are living. When it comes to managing your life after cancer, when treatment is completed, it can help to redefine your whole life, as daunting as that sounds. Take adequate time to think, write, and talk about what your "new normal" life looks like, exploring this idea as it relates to your body (what you can do to keep it well), your mind (how you are thinking differently about your life, what thoughts sustain you and nourish you now), your heart (how you take care of yourself emotionally when you fear a recurrence, and how you let others love you in new ways now), and your spirit (how you think and feel differently about God and spirituality in your life after treatment is done). A "new normal" life is made up of what has changed because of the cancer, and includes what you have lost as a result of cancer, what you have gained as a result of cancer, what you are choosing to let go of as a result of cancer, and what you are choosing to let in now, as a result of cancer.

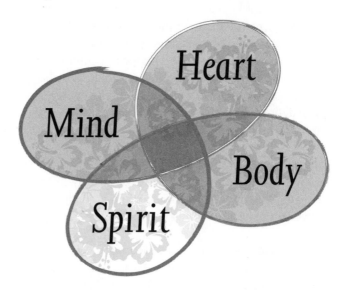

Breast Cancer And Your Spirit:
The Ways You Think And Feel About God
And Your Spirituality

"Why did God give me this cancer?"

"Breast cancer blew my spirit open. It made me embrace what I already knew, but be it and think it more, thankfully. I

know I'm not alone, ever."

"I've never been religious or spiritual. It was never part of my upbringing. But I don't know where to turn to inside myself now."

"What can I count on and control? The love I give and receive. I can take that for granted when everything else is falling apart."

"Before, I was angry at God for my early life. I stopped being angry at God when I got cancer."

"Cancer is like the holocaust, or the tsunami. God wasn't mad at all those people who died."

"I get restless in church for the first time in my life. I used to love it. It feels meaningless to me now, and I don't know why. That scares me. I've lost God."

"My mind likes to take control, and then connection to my spirit feels lost. Cancer has forced me inside, into this moment. Then I can find myself again."

"It's awful. My life was focused on my healthy lifestyle. I felt invincible. Cancer can happen anyway, to anyone. How can anybody feel safe, ever? If this can happen, anything can go wrong."

"My grandmother used to tell me, 'Security is knowing that we have none, except for God'. It confused me, but I never forgot. I think I finally understand what she meant by that."

"I'm still looking for spiritual tools. I want a connection with God on a more consistent basis, every day. No matter what I'm facing I want to have a sense of peace about it. I pray for peace."

"When I'm scared I'm trying to lean toward my wisdom instead of my fear."

"Cancer has helped me spiritually. I liked things to be the way I wanted them to be, before. Now I can let things just be the way they are. It's a more peaceful way to live. I could never figure out how to be this way, until now."

"I envy my friends who have what they call 'faith'. When there is nowhere to look, where do I look?"

"I learned how to fight, and hang on, and find solutions along the way. But now I'm told it's time to call Hospice. How can I let go of all I've learned and let myself die?"

"If I don't stop trying to control what I can't control—the cancer—and resent it, and be angry at it, I'll never heal into the kind of person I want to become. I want something good to come out of this whether I make it out alive or not."

"I'm trying to forgive myself for wasting the gifts I was given in this life. I could have done more, made more of an impact."

"I learned very well to get through years of cancer fears by living one day at a time, looking only at the small picture of what was immediately demanded of me. Now it seems I have to say goodbye and look at the big picture again. That is hard to do. Where am I going?"

"My wife and I look at the circle of life. Dying goes on every minute of every day, everywhere. It's normal and natural. It's easy to see that in nature. That comforts me."

Tips For The Journey:

In our lives, we all face three sets of lessons that teach us wisdom: the lessons of the dark (learning to let go of thoughts and beliefs that no longer fit or are hurtful to ourselves, and learning to feel whole in solitude), lessons of light (learning to let love in and hold on to it, walking through the fire that burns away our defenses, allowing for the depth and joy of emotional and spiritual intimacy) and lessons of the gray (learning to simply wait when we have already leaped into mid-air, relinquishing what no longer works well, but haven't yet landed at the next level of understanding or peace. This is practicing spiritual patience, and it's one of the most difficult tasks of all.)

It is common for people who are facing a trauma or crisis with no quick resolution to feel lost in the wilderness of their experience, beyond the reach of God. This can happen even as belief in God and in the power of God's love remain clear and strong. The feelings of loss and the impulse to justify the loss with thoughts of cancer as punishment can be devastating. What may be true instead is that when we fall off a cliff, so to speak, and are in a deeper, darker place than we've ever known, we need to do the important work of allowing God to find us. God seeks us, just as we seek God. Again, this can be a time of waiting, and the work is learning spiritual patience.

Many people do not consider themselves religious, or even spiritual. If this is true for you, it might help to define, clarify and focus on which values mean the most to you, and the beliefs that have sustained you throughout your life. How have you used these values to guide your choices during difficult experiences in the past? What have you learned about yourself having survived past crises? What gives your life meaning now? Where do you find hope now?

If the idea of faith is new and appealing, talk with people whose faith you admire, whose faith guides the choices they make. Let them be the first of many teachers.

When you feel most afraid or disheartened, what do you need to remember? What spiritual beliefs can you lean into now? Close your eyes and softly allow them to hold you, surround you, and fill you with peace. Allow all of the stress and anxiety to flow through you, going on its way without you. Become the boulder in the river of fear.

What are you praying for? Many people find their prayers changing as they move through the experience of cancer.

From prayers of pleading and longing, based upon fears, they find themselves simply asking for strength to move to the next step, trust to help manage fear, or the wisdom to allow the journey to take the path it needs to take, and the time it requires. Some simply ask for help.

Do you pray for yourself? Many people do not, and consider doing so to be selfish. Yet, when it comes to our spiritual health, we need to ask for what we want, and open to the answers as they come. You may become more comfortable seeking on your own behalf if you allow yourself to ask for qualities you need to be able to grow spiritually through the experience of cancer. For example: "Please help me to always feel Your presence in my heart...teach me to feel the peace I know is there, waiting behind my fears...fill me with trust in those who are working to make me better...give me patience and tolerance to bear this vulnerability...". Then you need to become aware of these qualities coming alive inside you. Asking is only half of the process.

Some say that prayer is speaking with God, while meditation is listening to God. You might decide to meditate. Mindfulness Meditation, practiced daily for 8 weeks, has been shown on MRIs to increase the amount of brain matter in the part of the brain where we manage fears. Such a practice trains our brains to let go of frightening thoughts, so they are no longer as capable of "kidnapping" our minds. Meditation teaches us to bring our attention to the present moment, when our lives can feel safe. It is the forethought of loss that causes us to worry.

When it comes time to die, we prepare ourselves. Hospice workers consistently hear patients say things that reflect a growing peace about letting go of this precious life, beloved families and loved ones, and work left unfinished. We somehow come to understand, when it is time to move on, that we have left enough of a legacy behind, that the energy of our passion for life is palpable and available for those we are leaving, and it is enough. How can this happen? Perhaps it is because we finally learn that being, when we can no longer do, illuminates an enhancement of our life energy, not a diminishment.

In Summary...

Learning to live and thrive with breast cancer requires that you focus on all the parts of your life—how you act, how you think, how you feel, and how you let yourself be loved— so that you can flow through this life altering experience, and arrive at a better place afterward, knowing your ability to heal and your own wholeness more deeply than you ever knew them before. For your body: rest, exercise, massage (with an oncology trained massage therapist), guided imagery (which is a journey inside your mind which can positively impact your body) yoga, acupuncture, relaxing breathing techniques and other complementary services can help. For your mind: cognitive behavioral therapy, family therapy, and seeking the guidance of those who have walked this path before you can diminish much of the stress. For your heart: emotional support, learning to cast a loving eye on yourself, family therapy, and seeking the wisdom of the wisest people you know, and the guidance of those who have been there, can help create your new path. For your spirit: prayer, consultations with spiritual teachers, developing a meditation practice, and silent retreats may illuminate the way ahead.

Because of the cancer, you and the people you love have been forced to consider the possibility of your death earlier than any of you would have thought necessary. As difficult and frightening as this is, it is also a gift. As you consider coming to terms with dying, you gain the wisdom of this journey earlier, and it can have an intentional positive impact on your own future and on the future of everyone who loves you. However you choose to move forward, encouraging yourself to fight the cancer and not yourself, and allowing yourself to receive in all of the ways mentioned above, will make a difference in both the quality of your journey now, and the feelings of peace which await.

Resources:

Kitchen Table Wisdom: Stories that Heal by Rachel Naomi Remen, MD

When The Heart Waits by Sue Monk Kidd

Invisble Heroes by Belleruth Naperstek

Hollis Sigler's Breast Cancer Journal with text by Susan Love, MD and James Yood

The Anxiety and Phobia Workbook by Edmund Bourne, PhD

Comfortable With Uncertainty by Pema Chodron

Grace For Each Hour: Through The Breast Cancer Journey by Mary J. Nelson

The Places That Scare You by Pema Chodron

The Wisdom of No Escape by Pema Chodron

Final Gifts by Maggie Callanan and Patricia Kelley

Internet Resources:

healthjourneys.com for powerful, tested, guided imagery CDs. Use your mind to impact your body in helpful ways.

wellspouse.org

American Cancer Society

Inspire.com

caringbridge.com

helpinghands.com

pandora.com (radio): Calm Meditation music

For Children:

Help Me Say Goodbye: Activities for Helping Kids Cope When a Special Person Dies

Nana Upstairs, Nana Downstairs by Tomi dePaola

Tear Soup by Schwiebert, DeKlyen, and Bills

The Hope Tree by Laura Numeroff and Wendy S. Harpham, MD

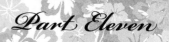

Part Eleven

Your Cancer Journal

YOUR WORKBOOK TO
COLLECT INFORMATION

Date of my diagnosis with cancer?_____

What type of cancer do I have?_____

Where did it start? _____

Has it spread to any other areas?_____

Where has it spread? _____

What is my cancer stage?_____

T _____ N _____ M _____

What are my current medications and doses?

1. _____
2. _____
3. _____
4. _____

I am allergic to these medications:

1. _____
2. _____
3. _____

What treatment have my health care providers recommended?

Surgery? _____

Radiation? _____
(Type and for how long)

Chemotherapy? _____
(Type and for how long)

Who are the care providers on my team? (Phone #)

1. _____
2. _____
3. _____
4. _____
5. _____

Record questions to be asked:

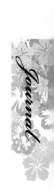

_____

_____

_____

_____

_____

_____

_____

_____

_____

_____

_____

_____

_____

_____

_____

_____

_____

_____

_____

_____

_____

_____

_____

_____

_____

_____

_____

_____

_____

_____

_____

_____

_____

_____

_____

_____

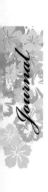

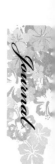

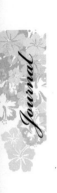

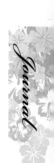

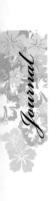

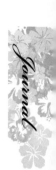

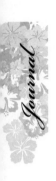

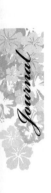

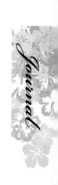

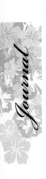

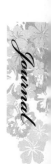

Notes and drawings:

Record dates and times of new symptoms for your records:

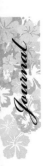

New Symptoms	Date And Time	Severity (1-10)

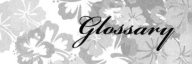

Common Cancer Terms

Adenocarcinoma: Cancer that originates from the glandular tissue of the breast.

Adjuvant therapy: Treatment used in addition to the main form of therapy. It usually refers to treatment utilized after surgery. As an example, chemotherapy or radiation may be given after surgery to increase the chance of cure.

Angiogenesis: The process of forming new blood vessels. Some cancer therapies work by blocking angiogenesis, and this blocks nutrients from reaching cancer cells.

Antigen: A substance that triggers an immune response by the body. This immune response involves the body making antibodies.

Benign tumor: An abnormal growth that is not cancer and does not spread to other areas of the body.

Biopsy: The removal of a sample of tissue to detect whether cancer is present.

Brachytherapy: Internal radiation treatment given by placing radioactive seeds or pellets directly in the tumor or next to it.

Cancer: The process of cells growing out of control due to mutations in DNA.

Carcinoma: A malignant tumor (cancer) that starts in the lining layer of organs. The most frequent types are lung, breast, colon, and prostate.

Chemotherapy: Medicine usually given by an IV or in pill form to stop cancer cells from dividing and spreading.

Clinical Trials: Research studies that allow testing of new treatments or drugs and compare the outcomes to standard treatments. Before the new treatment is studied on patients, it is studied in the laboratory. The human studies are called clinical trials.

Computerized Axial Tomography: Otherwise known as a CT scan. This is a picture taken to evaluate the anatomy of the body in three dimensions.

Cytokine: A product of the immune system that may stimulate immunity and cause shrinkage of some cancers.

Deoxyribonucleic Acid: Otherwise known as DNA. The genetic blueprint found in the nucleus of the cell. The DNA holds information on cell growth, division, and function.

Enzyme: A protein that increases the rate of chemical reactions in living cells.

Feeding tube: A flexible tube placed in the stomach through which nutrition can be given.

Gastro Esophageal Reflux Disease (GERD): A condition in which stomach acid moves up into the esophagus and causes a burning sensation.

Genetic Testing: Tests performed to determine whether someone has certain genes which increase cancer risk.

Grade: A measurement of how abnormal a cell looks under a microscope. Cancers with more abnormal appearing cells (higher grade tumors) have the tendency to be faster growing and have a worse prognosis.

Hereditary Cancer Syndrome: Conditions that are associated with cancer development and can occur in family members because of a mutated gene.

Histology: A description of the cancer cells which can distinguish what part of the body the cells originated from.

Immunotherapy: Treatments that promote or support the body's immune system response to a disease such as cancer.

Intensity Modulated Radiation Therapy: Also known as IMRT. A complex type of radiation therapy where many beams are used. It spares surrounding normal tissues and treats the cancer with more precision.

Leukemia: Cancer of the blood or blood-forming organs. People with leukemia often have a noticeable increase in white blood cells (leukocytes).

Localized cancer: Cancer that has not spread to another part of the body.

Lymph nodes: Bean shaped structures that are the "filter" of the body. The fluid that passes through them is called lymph fluid and filters unwanted materials like cancer cells, bacteria, and viruses.

Malignant: A tumor that is cancer.

Metastasis: The spread of cancer cells to other parts of the body such as the lungs or bones.

Monoclonal Antibodies: Antibodies made in the lab to work as homing devices for cancer cells.

Mutation: A change in the DNA of a cell. Cancer is caused by mutations in the cell which lead to abnormal growth and function of the cell.

Neoadjuvant therapy: Systemic and/or radiation treatment given before surgery to shrink a tumor.

Palliative treatment: Treatment that relieves symptoms, such as pain, but is not expected to cure the disease. Its main purpose is to improve the patient's quality of life.

Pathologist: A doctor trained to recognize tumor cells as benign or cancerous.

Positron Emission Tomography: Also known as a PET scan. This test is used to look at cell metabolism to recognize areas in the body where the cancer may be hiding.

Radiation therapy: Invisible high energy beams that can shrink or kill cancer cells.

Recurrence: When cancer comes back after treatment.

Remission: Partial or complete disappearance of the signs and symptoms of cancer. This is not necessarily a cure.

Risk factors: Environmental and genetic factors that increase our chance of getting cancer.

Side effects: Unwanted effects of treatment such as hair loss, burns or rash on the skin, sore throat, etc.

Simulation: Mapping session where radiation is planned. If the doctor will be using a mask for your treatment, this is the time it will be custom fit for your face.

Staging: Tests that help to determine if the cancer has spread to lymph nodes or other organs.

Standard Therapy: The most commonly used and widely accepted form of treatment that has been tested and proven.

Targeted Therapy: Modern cancer treatments that attack the part of cancer cells that make them different from normal cells. Targeted agents tend to have different side effects than conventional chemotherapy drugs.

Tumor: A new growth of tissue which forms a lump on or inside the body that may or may not be cancerous.

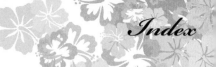
Index

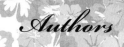

About The Authors

Stephanie R. Moline, MD, FACS: Dr. Moline is a Surgical Oncologist and Breast Surgeon at Cancer Care Northwest in Spokane, WA. She received her MD at Vanderbilt University in Nashville, TN in 1994 and fulfilled a residency and internship in surgery at the University of South Alabama in Mobile, AL from 1994-1999. She participated in a Fellowship for Breast Surgical Oncology at the University of Michigan in Ann Arbor, MI from 1999-2000.

Dr. Moline received special training in all aspects of breast surgery, particularly multi-disciplinary team care and advanced training in accelerated partial breast irradiation. She is skilled in office-based ultrasounds, same-day breast biopsy, as well as genetics and high risk breast cancer management.

Dr. Moline is certified by the American Board of Surgery and is a Fellow at the American College of Surgeons. She is also a member of the Spokane County Medical Society, a Research and Education Committee member of the American Society of Breast Surgeons, the National Surgical Adjuvant Breast Project, and the American Society of Breast Disease.

Since joining Cancer Care Northwest in 2002, Dr. Moline has greatly contributed to her passion of educating people about breast cancer and cancer-related topics.

Joni Nichols, MD: Dr. Nichols is originally from upstate New York. She attended Dartmouth College, graduating magna cum laude with a degree in Biochemistry. She received her MD from Duke University in 1985. She subsequently completed her internal medicine residency at University of California, San Francisco, including one year of Chief Residency. She began her Hematology/Oncology Fellowship at UCLA and completed her training at Stanford University.

She moved to Spokane with her family in 1993 and joined Cancer Care NW as the sixth medical oncologist in 1995. Over the years her practice has evolved to primarily caring for breast cancer patients.

She also has a strong interest in palliative care and has been a medical director of Hospice of Spokane since 1996.

Victor Gonzalez, MD: Dr. Gonzales is a Board Certified Radiation Oncologist and Assistant Professor at the University of Arizona Cancer Center. He specializes in radiotherapy for breast cancer and lymphoma.

Dr. Gonzalez completed his undergraduate training at the University of Florida where he graduated with highest honors. He earned his medical degree from Florida State University where he was elected to the AOA medical honor society. After completing his internship in internal medicine at the University of California San Diego, he trained in Radiation Oncology at the University of Utah's Huntsman Cancer Institute where he served as Chief Resident. He is a member of the RTOG and SWOG cooperative oncology groups. Dr. Gonzalez is a member of the American Society of Radiation Oncology, the American Society of Clinical Oncology and the American Association for the Advancement of Science.

Dr. Gonzalez has published research in peer-reviewed journals and has presented his findings at national research conferences. His work includes investigation of innovative techniques for breast radiotherapy as well as methods for improving intensity modulated radiation therapy. His current areas of research include advanced treatment modalities for radiation therapy following mastectomy and methods for reducing short and long term side effects from breast radiotherapy.

Saritha Thumma, MD: Dr. Thumma is originally from Hyderabad, a city in southern India. She graduated from St. John's Medical College, where she received her MD in 2000. She subsequently completed her internal medicine residency at the Medical College of Wisconsin in Milwaukee. On completing her residency, she attended the University of Minnesota and commenced her Hematology/Oncology Fellowship.

After finishing her fellowship, she moved to Spokane in 2010 to join Cancer Care Northwest, a multi-disciplinary oncology practice. Her primary interest is in thoracic malignancies, with a special emphasis in treating breast cancer patients. She participates actively in clinical trials.

Dr. Thumma is board certified in Internal Medicine and Medical Oncology.

Robert K. Fairbanks, MD: Dr. Fairbanks is the son of an Educator/Sculptor from

Southeastern Arizona. His undergraduate studies were in cell biology at Arizona State University. During his undergraduate studies, he was awarded two patents for work in semiconductor research. From 1988 to 1992, he attended Tulane University School of Medicine in New Orleans during which time he was awarded research grants from the American Heart and the American Diabetes Associations. During Medical School he completed a two month Lymphoma Research assignment at the Mayo Clinic. After Graduation from medical school, he served as Chief Resident and completed his internship in the transitional residency program at Tulane Medical Center. His Radiation Oncology residency training was completed at Johns Hopkins Hospital in Baltimore where he again served a year as Chief Resident. He then took a position as an Associate Professor of Radiation Oncology with Texas A&M Medical School. Subsequently he practiced Radiation Oncology in Everett, WA and now is with Cancer Care Northwest a multi-disciplinary Cancer Clinic in Spokane, WA.

He is a Board Certified in Therapeutic Radiology/Radiation Oncology. He has interest in clinical research, and has co-authored multiple scientific articles. He has special interest in intracranial and body radiosurgery & intraoperative radiotherapy/brachytherapy. He maintains outside interest in art, travel and scuba diving.

Wayne T. Lamoreaux, MD: Dr. Lamoreaux, was born in Southern California and spent his formative years in Arizona. After graduating magna cum laude from Utah State University in 1996, he completed medical school at the University of Utah in 2000, and then fulfilled a one year internship in Spokane Washington. In 2005, he finished a four year Radiation Oncology Residency at Washington University in St. Louis, where he served as Chief Resident, and was awarded the RSNA Roentgen Resident/Fellow Research Award. He is a board-certified Radiation Oncologist and current President of Cancer Care Northwest, a regionally comprehensive, multi-specialty oncology physician group located in Spokane, Washington. They run four integrated cancer centers and seven outreach clinics throughout the Inland Northwest.

Throughout his career, he has maintained leadership and research interests aimed at improving the treatment and the outcome of patients with cancer. He has co-authored multiple scientific articles and book chapters and presented his work at national and international meetings. He is married with four children, is fluent in Spanish, and enjoys soccer, snow skiing and water sports.

Jason A. Call, MD: Dr. Call attended Brigham Young University where he graduated cum laude in 2003 with a double major in Zoology and Russian. He received an M.D. in 2007 from the Medical College of Wisconsin. He participated in a summer research fellowship in the Department of Radiation Oncology during his medical school education. After completing an internship year at Aurora St. Luke's Medical Center, he went on to receive four more years of training in Radiation Oncology at the Mayo Clinic in Rochester, MN. He also has special training in Gynecologic Brachytherapy that was completed at the American Brachytherapy Society School of GYN Brachytherapy in Chicago, IL.

Throughout his career Dr. Call has been active in clinical oncology research. He has presented his research at national and international oncology meetings, published scientific papers in peer reviewed journals, and has published chapters for Oncology textbooks. He joined Cancer Care Northwest as a Radiation Oncologist in 2012.

Heather Gabbert, MS, RD, LD, CD: Heather attended Southern Illinois University at Carbondale and graduated with her Master's Degree in Dietetics in 1995. She has been a Registered Dietitian (RD) for 17 years and has lived in different areas of the country throughout the years, in each place, gaining valuable experience in the field of dietetics. She has worked with cancer patients since 1998 when she began working at Cancer Treatment Centers of America. She continued to work intermittently for CTCA throughout the many years she has been a practitioner. Heather moved to Spokane, Washington, from Chicago, Illinois, in 2007 where she works as an RD for Cancer Care Northwest and a home health company. Professionally, Heather's passion lies in working with cancer patients and promoting wellness and disease prevention for all.

Heather is a member of Academy of Nutrition and Dietetics (AND), Washington State Academy of Nutrition and Dietetics (WSAND), and Greater Spokane Dietetics Association (GSDA). She served for two years as Media Representative and board member for WSAND and GSDA. Heather has authored a book, been a contributing writer, written articles and was a blogger for StepUpSpokane, highlighting nutrition and wellness. She is a member of AND's DPG groups: Oncology, Business Communications and Entrepreneurs, Dietitians in Integrative Medicine, and Sports, Cardio and Wellness Nutrition (SCAN) group.

Heather most enjoys time spent with her two children. She also enjoys life as a Zumba instructor, exerciser and most memorable activities are her first half marathon and participating in an adventure race, which involved trail-running, biking and kayaking.

Tess Taft, MSW, LICSW: Tess is an oncology stress management specialist and family therapist who has served cancer patients and their loved ones in hospitals, cancer clinics, homes, nursing homes, hospices and private practice settings for 34 years. She received a Masters Degree in Social Work from The University of Washington in 1979 and completed a Marriage and Family Therapy training program in 1981. In 1990 she became a certified specialist in Interactive Guided Imagery for Medical Clinicians in order to teach clients this unique and powerful tool to help with symptom and stress management, and to explore and deepen hope and faith. She has taught a Palliative Care certification program for graduate social work students at Eastern Washington University since 2007, which includes 3 classes: Family Systems and Illness, Death and Dying, and Alternatives in Healing. Tess has provided trainings nationally, as well as clinical supervision for many therapists over the years. She is committed to serving people whose life-threatening diagnosis, or that of a love, has propelled them on a journey inside themselves to find emotional and spiritual healing and peace.

Kathy Beach, RN: Kathy graduated with her RN degree in 1993. She decided to get a degree in nursing after her mother was diagnosed with breast cancer. She spent sixteen years in hospital nursing where she worked on a wide range of units from Medical Oncology to Outpatient Surgery. For the past 4 years, she has focused her energy in oncology and radiation oncology with Cancer Care Northwest in Spokane, WA. She loves her work and finds the patients she cares for and their families to be extremely inspiring.

Christopher M. Lee, MD: Dr. Lee is a practicing Radiation Oncologist and is the Director of Research for Cancer Care Northwest and The Gamma Knife of Spokane (Spokane, WA). Dr. Lee graduated cum laude in Biochemistry from Brigham Young University in 1997 which included a summer research fellowship at Harvard University and Brigham and Women's Hospital. He subsequently attended Saint Louis University School of Medicine where he received his M.D. with Distinction in Research degree. He completed four additional years of specialty training in Radiation Oncology at the Huntsman Cancer Hospital and University of Utah Medical Center. Dr. Lee has actively pursued both basic science and clinical research throughout his career. He continues to publish scientific papers and give presentations on radiotherapy technique and the use of targeted radiation in the care of patients with head and neck (throat), brain, breast, gynecologic, and prostate malignancies.

This patient handbook is the breast cancer volume of the "Living And Thriving With..." series.

We greatly appreciate the educational grant by:

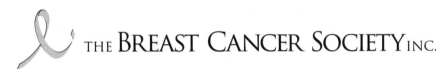

THE BREAST CANCER SOCIETY INC.

which largely funded the development of this patient-centered guidebook.

We also express appreciation to:

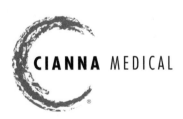

CIANNA MEDICAL

whose grant helped fund this patient-centered guidebook.